Palliative Day Care

HOSPICE CARE FOR BURNLEY & PENDLE
Pendleside   Colne Road   Reedley
BURNLEY   BB10 2LW
Tel: 01282 440100   FAX: 01282 601735

Palliative Day Care

Edited by

Ronald A Fisher MA, MRCS, LRCP, FRCA
Lecturer in Palliative Care and formerly Consultant
Physician in Palliative Medicine,
Macmillan Unit, Christchurch Hospital, Dorset, UK

and

Pearl McDaid SRN, NDN Cert, FETC, PWT
Former Senior Nurse, Day Care Services,
Michael Sobell House, Dept of Palliative Medicine,
Mount Vernon Hospital, Northwood, Middlesex, UK
Chairman of the National Association of Hospice/Palliative
Day Care Leaders

Preface by

G W Hanks BSc, FRCP, FRCPE, FFPM
Professor of Palliative Medicine, University of Bristol Oncology
Centre, Bristol, UK

A member of the Hodder Headline Group
LONDON • SYDNEY • AUCKLAND

First published in Great Britain 1996 by
Arnold, a member of the Hodder Headline group,
338 Euston Road, London NW1 3BH

Whilst the advice and information in this book is believed to be true and
accurate at the date of going to press, neither the editors, authors nor the publisher
can accept any legal responsibility or liability for any errors or omissions
that may be made. In particular (but without limiting the generality of the
preceding disclaimer) every effort has been made to check drug dosages;
however it is still possible that errors have been missed. Furthermore,
dosage schedules are constantly being revised and new side-effects
recognised. For these reasons the reader is strongly urged to consult the
drug companies' printed instructions before administering any of the drugs
recommended in this book.

British Library Cataloguing in Publication Data
A catalogue record for this book is available from the British Library

Library of Congress Cataloging-in-Publication Data
A catalog record for this book is available from the Library of Congress

ISBN 0 340 62521 X

Typeset in 10/11pt Ehrhardt
Printed and bound in Great Britain by J. W. Arrowsmith Ltd, Bristol

Contents

Preface

Modern palliative care began just over a quarter of a century ago with the opening of St Christopher's Hospice in London. This marked a fundamental change in approach to the management of incurable illness and dying patients and has had a worldwide impact. As the pioneers repeatedly emphasised in those early days, hospice, or palliative, care is not about bricks and mortar or about care that can take place only in a particular type of building or physical environment. Rather it is a philosophy of care which focuses on the patient rather than the illness, and which recognises the unit of care as the patient *and his or her family.* Early in the evolution of palliative care came the recognition of the need for services to take such care into the patient's home. A working group of a government advisory committee recommended in 1980 that terminal care for cancer should be based at home, and that 'an integrated system of care should be developed with emphasis on coordination between the primary care sector, the hospital sector and the hospice movement'. The same report urged that terminal care units should explore 'the advantages of day care'.

The first day hospice was described by Wilkes and his colleagues in 1978. Since then there has been an enormous increase in the number of such services, which now exceeds that of in-patient palliative care and hospice units. This strategy of giving priority to home care and day care has been endorsed by successive reports on palliative care provision in the UK. The National Association of Health Authorities, in their 1987 guidelines on standards and services for terminally ill people, recommended that the development of specialist nursing services and day care should have priority over in-patient provision. The most recent report of the government's standing medical and nursing advisory committees (1992) recommends that 'palliative care services are integrated with general practice'.

Given this background and increasing emphasis on day care it is surprising to discover that there is very little written about this area of palliative care. A recent survey conducted by Help the Hospices highlights considerable variations in accommodation and staffing, and other resources such as transport and volunteer services. This situation reflects the dearth of published information or guidance on the setting up and running of such services. This book is designed to fill this gap in the palliative care literature. Ronnie Fisher and Pearl McDaid have brought together much experience and wisdom to aid and guide those planning day care services. The book is based on experience in the UK, but as with other aspects of palliative care this approach and philosophy will be just as applicable in many other cultures and environments.

There is still much to be achieved. In spite of the emphasis on terminal care at home, and in spite of the fact that most patients with advanced cancer express a wish to die at home, the proportion of home deaths from cancer in the UK is actually declining and is currently about 25 per cent. I have no doubt that day care has a fundamental role to play in supporting patients and families at home, and that wider provision of such facilities will remain a priority for some time to come. I have no doubt also that this book will provide a valuable resource for those attempting to meet this need.

GW Hanks 1996

List of contributors

Caroline Badger BA, RGN
Macmillan Nurse Consultant in Lymphoedema, Oxford, UK

Rita Benor RGN, RHV, RM, DN Cert, RNT, Cert Ed, M BAFATT, Cert Counselling
Lecturer in Palliative Care and Psychotherapist, Psychotherapist, Autogenic Training Therapist, South Devon, UK

Jo Bray DipCOT, SROT
Head, Occupational Therapist, Warren Pear! Marie Curie Centre, Solihull, West Midlands, UK

Bruce Driver LLB, FCIS, Dip Theol
Honorary Chaplain, Michael Sobell House, Mount Vernon Hospital, Northwood, Middlesex, UK

Ronald A Fisher MA, MRCS, LRCP, FRCA
Lecturer in Palliative Care and formerly Consultant Physician in Palliative Medicine, Macmillan Unit, Christchurch Hospital, Dorset, UK

Lydia Gillham BA, MCSP, SRP, Dip TP
Director of Educational Development and Senior Physiotherapist, St Oswald's Hospice, Gosforth, Newcastle upon Tyne, UK

G W Hanks BSc, FRCP, FRCPE, FFPM
Professor of Palliative Medicine, University of Bristol Oncology Centre, Bristol, UK

Irene Higginson BMedSci, BM BS, MFPHM, PhD
Senior Lecturer and Consultant, London School of Hygiene and Tropical Medicine, University of London, London, UK

Jo Hockley RGN, SCM, MSc
Clinical Nurse Specialist in Palliative Care, Western General Hospital, Edinburgh, UK

Tim Hunt MD, DSc, MRCP
Consultant Physician in Palliative Medicine, Arthur Rank House, Brookfields Hospital, Cambridge, UK

Gavin Jenkins MA, DipCOT, SROT
Senior Occupational Therapist, Mary Marlborough Centre, Oxford, UK

David Johnson DMS, MMS (Dip)
Chief Executive, St Mary's Hospice, Birmingham, UK

Ian Johnson
Community Relations Director, St Helena Hospice, Colchester, Essex, UK

Marian Longley Dip Counselling
Voluntary Services Manager, Hayward House, City Hospital, Nottingham, UK

Gillian Luff B SocSc, AIMSW
Macmillan Lecturer in Social Work and Palliative Care, Faculty of Business and
Social Studies, Cheltenham and Gloucester College of Higher Education,
Cheltenham, Gloucestershire, UK

Pearl McDaid SRN, NDN Cert, FETC, PWT
79 Elm Grove, Woburn Sands, Milton Keynes, Bedfordshire, UK
Former Senior Nurse, Day Care Services, Michael Sobell House, Dept of
Palliative Medicine, Mount Vernon Hospital, Northwood, Middlesex, UK.
Chairman, National Association of Hospice/Palliative Day Care Leaders

Veronica Moss MRCP, DTM&H
Medical Director, Mildmay Mission Hospital, London, UK

Mabel Mowatt BA, Cert Child Care
Day Hospice Coordinator, St Columbus Hospice, Edinburgh, UK

Shirley Parnis NNEB, CQSW, CGLI, Cert Counselling
Senior Social Worker, Social Services Department, Addenbrooke's Hospital,
Cambridge, UK

Jenny Penson MA(ed), SRN, HV, Cert Ed, RNT, Cert Counselling
Macmillan Nurse Tutor, North Devon Hospice Care Trust, Barnstaple, UK

Patrick Russell MB BS, DRCOG
Honorary Medical Advisor, Peace Hospice, Watford, Hertfordshire, UK and
formerly Family Physician and Hospital Practitioner, Michael Sobell House,
Mount Vernon Hospital, Northwood, Middlesex, UK

Derek Spooner MHSM, DipHSM, MBIM
Consultant Planning Adviser to Cancer Relief Macmillan Fund

Ann Stead DipCOT, SROT
Clinical Director, Rehabilitation Technology, Mary Marlborough Centre, Oxford,
UK

Sue Taylor SRN, SCM, HV Cert
Centre Manager, Neil Cliffe Cancer Centre, Wythenshawe Hospital, Manchester,
UK

Acknowledgements

Pioneers of the hospice movement have been described as enthusiastic amateurs. Since we are a rather young specialty some of those amateurs are still very much alive, while others alas, have passed on. Nevertheless this must have caused some wry amusement in this green and pleasant land and not a little derisory laughter in the Elyssian Fields. They can of course take solace in the knowledge that though the Titanic was built by professionals, amateurs built the Ark.

We take pleasure therefore in dedicating this book and paying tribute to those pioneering enthusiastic amateurs who, following in the footsteps of Dame Cicely Saunders, helped to lay the foundations of palliative care as we know it today.

Our contributors have a special excellence – they have something to say – and since 'the pen is the tongue of the hand' then without doubt they have said it well. To them we give our most sincere thanks.

Part I: Philosophy

1

Purpose

Ronald Fisher and Pearl McDaid

There is one quality more important than 'know-how'.
This is to 'know what' by which we determine not only
how to accomplish our purposes but what our purposes are to be.
                    Norbert Weiner, The Human Use of Human Beings (1954), 10

Our purpose in this book is to guide and advise individuals and organisations who wish to establish a palliative day care service, whether it be in a house converted for this purpose, in an unused ward that has been readapted, or in a specially designed (purpose built) free-standing unit. The scale of service can extend from that which is adequate to a comprehensive all-embracing programme that could be 'the hub' of a palliative care service for any area.

By collating information and expertise from our contributors we hope to provide a comprehensive guide which encompasses every aspect of day care.

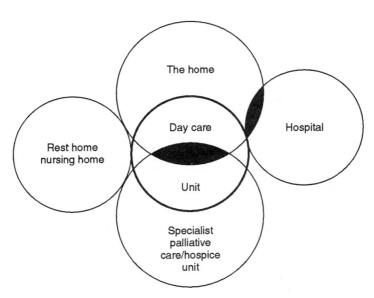

Fig. 1.1 A day care unit can be the hub for palliative care in the community.

The majority of those suffering from incurable and life-threatening illness wish to live and be cared for at home. While good symptom control and psychological support can be provided by professional carers in the community, there is often an urgent need for peer group support.

Professionals who work in palliative care are aware that for most patients the diagnosis and treatment of malignant disease is a devastating intrusion into their lives. For those patients whose disease is life threatening and incurable, many adjustments have to be made in their lifestyles. They are often too incapacitated to pursue their usual routines and hobbies, and quite often they and their families are left stunned by the situation. It is for those patients who are not actually dying, but whose ability to fulfil their usual roles is compromised, that referral to a day care unit is indicated.

Shirley Parnis writes (*see* Chapter 3) that one of the key objectives of the National Health Service and Community Care Act which became fully operational in April 1993 is to promote the development of domiciliary day care and respite services to enable people to live at home for as long as possible. This emphasis on care in the community means day care can become the spearhead of any palliative care programme.

It is anticipated that fewer in-patient hospices will be built in the immediate future. These, in any case, do not have the monopoly of providing clinical, educational and research expertise. These skills can be available within a hospice day care setting.

For the purpose of this book the expressions 'palliative care' and 'hospice care' have exactly the same meaning. However, this does not apply to that bleak phrase 'terminal care', which is no more than a part of palliative care[1] and lasts 'only a few days bringing new and more difficult problems'.[2]

The title 'palliative medicine' may not have received universal acceptance but as has so often been asked, 'what's in a name?' Shakespeare with devastating clarity provided the perfect answer:

What's in a name?
that which we call a rose
By any other name would smell as sweet.

That which we call palliative care would by any other name be just as caring.

So let us define what we mean by palliative care by using the World Health Organization definition:

The study and management of patients with active, progressive, far advanced disease for which the prognosis is limited and the focus of care is on the quality of life.

The World Health Organization later amplified this definition:

Palliative care affirms life and regards death as a normal process, neither hastens nor postpones death, provides relief from pain and other distressing symptoms, integrates the psychological and spiritual aspects of patient care and offers a support system to help the family cope during the patient's illness and in their bereavement.

Day care objectives

A summary of day care philosophy is appropriate at this stage and certain aspects will be highlighted in the following pages:

- Day care can be a continuing life line of support.
- It enables patients to remain at home and it is a haven for those who live alone.
- It focuses on the quality of life by attending to the physical, psychological, emotional, social and spiritual needs of patients and their families.
- It provides rehabilitation (*see* Chapter 2) in order to maximise self reliance, minimal dependency and promote confidence.
- It can provide social stimulus, eliminate boredom and iatrogenic isolation.
- It provides a change of environment.
- It can facilitate creativity and personal growth.
- It enables the patient's progress to be monitored.
- It is a vital source of respite care.

There is much untapped talent in the community and a palliative day care centre provides an opportunity for local people to participate in its activities.

Eric Wilkes[3] has rightly expressed the fear that if improved community services are able to delay admission into an in-patient bed until just before death, then that trusting relationship which is found in a hospice environment will not have had time to develop. This is a timely warning but there is no reason to doubt that 'the hospice soul' can still flourish in day care hospices and so trusting relationships will continue to develop.

Day care is an essential part of domiciliary care and they should complement each other.

To enable patients to die at home Thorpe summarises the basic needs[4]:

- adequate nursing care;
- a night sitting service;
- good symptom control;
- confident and committed general practitioners;
- access to specialist care;
- effective coordination of care;
- financial support;
- palliative care education.

To this list we would add a 'sitter service' for the day time (*see* Chapter 15), and a greater use of the fund of experience and wisdom of the district nursing service. Their expertise could be enhanced with further education and updating in palliative care. It seems that there has been a lack of opportunity here which has resulted in some de-skilling and disregard of the potential of a very worthy body of nurses.[5]

Over the following pages our contributors will focus on the many aspects that together constitute palliative day care. They will provide the 'know how'.

A planning philosophy, where to build, what should be provided, landscaping and costings are all discussed in detail. Likewise constructive guidance is given on management and administration; and public relations and fund raising.

In order to improve the quality of palliative day care, the urgent need of clinical audit, evaluation and outcome is stressed. There is advice on the services that can be provided in the various clinics, namely, consultations, counselling, lymphoedema chemotherapy, complementary medicine, stress management and information.

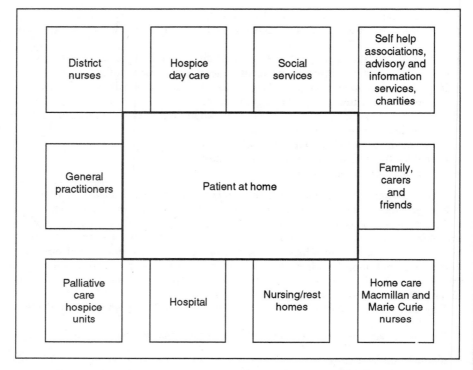

Fig. 1.2 Some sources of physical, psychological, social and financial help.

Staff requirements, not only medical and nursing, but the roles of the physio-therapist, the occupational therapist, the social worker, the chaplain and volun-teers are all described. It is crucial that those who work in this field pass on their knowledge and expertise, in order to enhance the skills of others, not only by in-house education but proactively.

The relentless progression of motor neurone disease (MND) is explained and we are told that the provision of palliative care for these patients is a relatively new concept. There are skills in a palliative day care setting that could be used to alleviate symptoms and to some extent 'compensate for or overcome some of the disability'.

The chapter on AIDS indicates the formidable difficulties that are to be faced when dealing with this disease. It is far from easy to draw the line between acute/active palliative treatment. It is important to understand the social, emotional and spiritual issues as well as the physical problems. Different models are described.

You can lead a patient to the table but you cannot always make him eat. A well-planned, gleamingly hygienic kitchen is not in itself sufficient to stimulate a patient's appetite. There has to be a therapeutic input as the chapter on nutri-tional hints indicates.

Finally, rehabilitation, which draws together so many of the above mentioned services, is the hub of palliative day care.

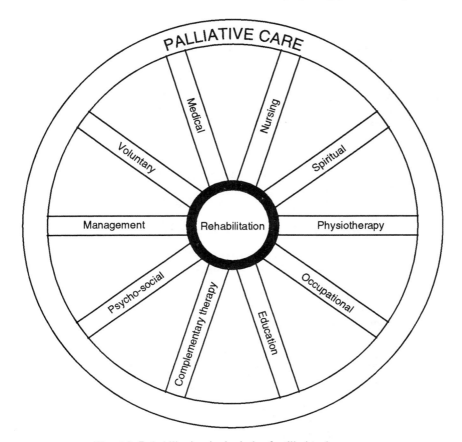

Fig. 1.3 Rehabilitation is the hub of palliative day care.

We are building in this book a comprehensive holistic base for as many services as possible.

Respite care

Respite care is an extremely important provision, because a common cause of admission to an in-patient bed is the inability of the principal carer or carers to cope with the stress and exhaustion of looking after a patient at home.

This is a distressing and devastating situation. The carer does not want to give in, and is overwhelmed by a feeling of guilt. The patient in all probability will understand, but the sadness will be there and there may even be a tinge of resentment.

However, domiciliary carers and specialists who are monitoring the patient's progress and the reactions of the family, may in many cases be able to anticipate such a crisis and either prevent it or delay its onset.

This means the referral to day care should not be delayed for too long, and attendances should be frequent enough, increased if necessary, to make it easier for the patient and the family to cope. It is unlikely that one attendance a week will be sufficient in the long run.

If you have to cut down attendances or turn away patients because of increasing demand, then you will be failing your community. This may be because of miscalculation initially, or insufficient funding that has resulted in your not building a big enough unit. I can only stress the importance of 'thinking big'.

There are other remedies that will help:

- We can move away from the 5-day week concept, and stay open at weekends. To a struggling family, a Saturday and Sunday can be just as stressful as any other day of the week.
- It may be possible to have smaller 'branch' units and if necessary patients can rotate with the parent centre.
- Night nursing and 'sitter' services also have a part to play.

Other specialties, whether oncology, radiotherapy or medical, should be aware of the benefits that palliative day care centres can offer and should be encouraged to use them.

Day care provides a day out for the patient and a day off for the carer. Obviously this is not all that day care services provide, but as the word 'respite' implies it provides a break, a lull, a breather, a rest, a holiday for the participants.

For a specified time the patient and the carer go their separate ways, therapeutic for one, a boon for the other and beneficial to both.

Bear in mind that it is highly probable that whatever you build will prove to be too small in the longer term. If you are planning for ten attendances a day in no time at all you will require space for fifteen places. This could mean another bathroom, another toilet, a larger dining area, more clinical space and so on. So think big!

Appendix

Table 1.1 Statistics on cancer

Worldwide
50 million people die from cancer every year throughout the world.
38 million in developing countries.
12 million in developed countries.

Three to four out of ten patients are cured in developed countries.
Fewer than two out of ten are cured in developing countries.

Europe
22% of all deaths are due to cancer.[6]

UK
25% of all deaths are due to cancer.
Over 300 000 new cases are registered each year;
70% of which are in-patients aged 60 years or more.

Population projections based on demographic trends suggest there is going to be a significant increase in the numbers of elderly people in the coming years. The statistics for cancer occurrence given in Table 1.1 are a good indication of the great need for palliative day care for patients with incurable and life-threatening disease.

Motor neurone disease

Sharon Barker, Information Service coordinator of the Motor Neurone Disease Association has kindly provided the national statistics for the UK.

Table 1.2 Statistics on motor neurone disease

The following statistics are based on information supplied by the Office of Population Censuses and Surveys.

Incidence
Incidence in England and Wales is approximately two cases per 100 000 people per year, similar to MS.

Prevalence
Owing to the rapid progression of MND, the prevalence is only about seven per 100 000 compared with about 50 per 100 000 for MS.
Number of deaths from MND

	1989	1990	1991	1992
Male	627	600	579	659
Female	533	576	506	559

This shows an increase since the 1980s in the number of people for whom MND was mentioned on the death certificate and a slight increase in the proportion of men. Current figures continue to show a slight increase, but whether this is due to more cases or better diagnosis is still unclear.

Proportion of total deaths
Approximately one in 450 of the people who die in England and Wales has MND. This is illustrated by the following figures for 1992:

	Total deaths	MND	Proportion
Female	286 600	530	1 in 513
Male	271 700	592	1 in 412

Comparison with other neurological diseases
This is a comparison between the number of deaths from MND and the number of deaths from other diseases. The numbers of deaths from each disease are ranked, using 1992 data:

Ranking for females:		Ranking for males:	
Alzheimer's	1320	Alzheimer's	691
MND	559	MND	659
MS	536	MS	260
Muscular dystrophy	73	Muscular dystrophy	170

August 1994

As far as she knows there are no equivalent international statistics. However, after discussions with members of the International Alliance of ALS/MND Associations, who between them represent most of the Americas, Europe and some of the Far East, there is a general feeling of the incidence and prevalence noted for the UK is broadly similar for their own areas.[7]

Aids and HIV

Epidemiological surveillance of the acquired immune deficiency syndrome (AIDS) started at the Public Health Laboratory Service Centre in collaboration with the Scottish centre in 1982.[8]

Surveillance of human immune deficiency virus (HIV) infection, the cause of AIDS, commenced in late 1984. Owing to the length and variability of the period between infection with HIV and development of AIDS (average of between 8 and 10 years), reports of AIDS cases do not give a picture of the current spread of HIV infection.

The results of HIV/AIDS forecasting by the World Health Organization should be considered conservative.[9]

Table 1.3 Statistics on HIV/AIDS

UK[8]
A total of 10 304 cases have been reported in the UK between 1982 and the end of December 1994.
    The number of AIDS cases reported in 1994 was 11% higher than in 1993.
    The cumulative total of recognised HIV infections is now 23 104.

January 20th 1995

Alzheimer's disease

An increase in Alzheimer's disease will be an inevitable by-product of an increase in the number of elderly people. This has major and social implications for the purchasers and suppliers of health and social services as the demand on financial and other resources increases.

Table 1.4 Age and prevalence of Alzheimer's disease in the UK

Age (years)	Prevalence
40–65	0.1% (1 in 1000)
65–70	2.0% (1 in 50)
70–80	5.0% (1 in 20)
80 plus	20% (1 in 5)

UK. It is currently estimated that there are 636 000 people with dementia in the UK, and of these nearly 500 000 will have Alzheimer's disease.[13] Over the next 30 years approximately 258 000 people will develop dementia, accounting for 894 000 people by the year 2021.

Worldwide. Alzheimer's disease affects more than 15 million persons worldwide.

Europe. Alzheimer's disease is the most chronic terminal illness among older people in the European Union affecting an estimated 3.5 million.

Table 1.5 Predictions for dementia in the UK

Age Year	0.1%* 40–64	2–5%* 65–79	20%* 80 plus	Total 40 plus	Total pop. 40 plus
1991	15 000	235 000	386 000	636 000	22.7 m
2001	16 000	235 000	454 000	704 000	24.5 m
2011	18 000	243 000	512 000	773 000	27.3 m
2021	17 000	304 000	572 000	894 000	28.3 m

*Prevalence.
Rough estimates based on OPCS Monitor PP2 93/1 February 1993

Table 1.6 Statistics on Parkinson's disease[10]

Parkinson's disease is found worldwide and studies suggest a crude prevalence of 1:1000 of the general population.
It is found predominately in old age.
In the UK, for example, where the incidence is also 1:1000 of the general population, it rises to:
    1:100 in those over 65 years and
    1:50 in those over 80 years.
A total of 120 000 people in the UK currently have the disease.[11, 12]
Many sufferers from Parkinson's disease are dependent on others for a wide range of activities.

References

1. Fisher R. Chapter 1 Introduction: Palliative care – a rediscovery. In: Penson J, Fisher R, eds *Palliative care for people with cancer.* London: Edward Arnold, 1995.
2. Saunders C. Some challenges that face us. *J Palliative Med* 1993; 7(2): 77–83.
3. Wilkes E. Introduction. In: Clark D, ed. *The future for palliative care.* Buckingham: Open University Press, 1993; 1–5.
4. Thorpe G. Enabling more dying people to remain at home. *BMJ* 1993; 307: 915–18.
5. Regnard C. Access to specialist palliative care. *BMJ* 1994; 308: 655.
6. Stjernswärd J. A global problem addressed. *Europ J Palliative Care* 1994; 1(1): 6 & 7.
7. Motor Neurone Disease Association, PO Box 246, Northampton NN1 2PR.
8. Public Health Laboratory Service, 61 Colindale Avenue, London NW9 5DF.
9. Global Programme in AIDS, The HIV/AIDS Pandemic 1994 Overview, World Health Organization, Geneva, Switzerland.

10. Parkinson's Disease Society, 22 Upper Woburn Place, London WC1H ORA.
11. The Parkinson Papers, Issue 2, 1990. Designed and produced by Franklin Scientific Projects, 516 Wandsworth Road, London SW8 3JK.
12. West R. *Parkinson's disease*, Office of Health and Economics, London, 1991.
13. Alzheimer's Disease Society, Gordon House, 10 Greencoat Place, London SW1P 1PH.

2

Rehabilitation

Jo Hockley and Mabel Mowatt

You're looking at a train, standing in a station. It may not be moving right now, but trains move. That's how trains are.

W. Nicholson, 'Shadowlands'[1]

Introduction

To talk about rehabilitation within the setting of the day hospice might at first glance appear to be paradoxical. Indeed, in suggesting that a person might be rehabilitated by attending a day hospice, one might be accused of using a euphemism or of 'pulling the wool' over their eyes'.

What do we really mean by rehabilitation within the remit of this book? Restoration, reintegration, re-education, or readjustment? In this chapter a closer look will be taken at a working definition of rehabilitation within the context of the day hospice. There will be an emphasis that affirms the quality of life in the broadest sense of the term. It will explore the importance of realistic hope despite failing health, giving consideration to issues such as re-establishing relationships, reintegrating people from the isolation of a terminal illness/collusion, affirming patients' self worth, humour, and trying to bring an element of control back into what is often seen as a 'runaway' situation.

One cannot change the final destination of our patients entering the hospice for day care; this would be impossible short of a miracle. However, what we can try to do is to influence the quality of that journey.

Defining 'rehabilitation' in relation to the day hospice

To the lay person who is suffering from, or caring for someone with advanced disease/metastatic cancer, it is important that we do not knowingly mislead their understanding of 'rehabilitation'. Rehabilitation is defined by the Oxford Dictionary as 'to restore to a previous condition'. This idea of restoration is emphasised by the medical profession's definition in the 1940s:

> ... any process other than medical or surgical treatment applied to an individual to prevent or reduce his loss of capacity and to restore him to the maximum possible degree of mental and physical ability in the shortest space of time after illness and injury; and in order to complete this, his reinstatement into constructive work as a useful and contented member of the community.[2]

Even within the context of a chronic condition, such as a spinal injury, rehabilitation is unlikely to restore, i.e. make new. Rehabilitation can perhaps reintegrate the person back into society or re-educate them to be able to feel a useful member of their community again. However, in the context of rehabilitation and the day hospice are restoration, reintegration, re-education appropriate definitions? I think not.

Some 25 years ago Dietz (1969)[3] detailed four rehabilitative stages in cancer patients, namely: preventative, restorative, supportive and palliative. The acknowledgement of rehabilitation alongside palliative care by Dietz at this time is very commendable. More recently, Dietz (1981)[4] states that 'the goal of rehabilitation for people with cancer is to improve the quality of life for maximum productivity with minimum dependence, regardless of life expectancy'. However, we would argue that there is a difference in relating rehabilitation while facing a diagnosis of cancer, and rehabilitation facing a progressive, far advanced cancer/disease. Yes, quality of life and minimum dependence are important issues in both the above situations, but the essence of 'hope' and 'time'[5] become much more focused when the patient and family are trying to cope with end-stage disease. Rehabilitation within the context of palliative care becomes a situation that is unlikely to remain static for more than a few weeks at a time. We would like to suggest the following definition of rehabilitation in palliative care – one which, in many ways, re-emphasises hospice philosophy:

> The skilled help given to enable a person and their family to re-adjust to a situation that is unlikely to remain static for more than a few weeks at a time, because of progressive, far-advanced disease. Such help involves not only the expert control of distressing physical symptoms, but the exploration of strengths/coping strategies in relation to the patient's emotional/psychological/spiritual health. The outcome of such assistance alongside specialist therapies is designed to effect positively the quality of life, making the time lived worthwhile.

Quality of life may well vary from one person to another. What brings quality to one person's situation may well not be what adds quality to someone else's. None the less, life has to be worth living, even within the confines of a terminal illness; often it is 'others' that can influence this quality.

Quality of life

Quality of life is an abstract and complex term representing individual responses to the physical, mental and social factors which contribute to normal daily living.[6] The threat of death hanging over someone can in itself inevitably affect the quality of the life to be lived.[7] So often all a person facing a terminal illness asks for is to be able to carry out normal daily living activities. When this is not possible, powerlessness, loss of control and lack of choice are just a few of the factors that can undermine efforts to boost morale.

Patterson (1975)[8] details eight factors that contribute to the overall quality of life experience (*see* Figure 2.1). At first glance this list may not appear relevant within the day hospice situation; however, in helping our patients to adjust their goals, most of these factors then do take on a significance – a significance that can make a difference. For example: the 'personal satisfaction' in being able to complete a task however small; 'comparing oneself with others' facing a similar situation and seeing them have courage, and even a smile, can help to encourage the weakest psyche; 'being able to get symptoms under control' in order to enable the maximum level of functioning possible within the limits of the disease.

Perhaps one of the main factors that often needs addressing is that of self esteem. Patients who have been chronically ill and who have undergone many different treatments often feel guilty about being ill and a burden, not only to their families but to their friends and even society. They feel undervalued and their self esteem is often at rock bottom. It often requires enormous tact to gently work through the layers of self defence that have been used to try and protect the fragile ego. Poor communication in the family just compounds such a situation and often day hospice patients might find the rehabilitative team easier to talk to than their own family. This is not to say that the family is excluded. Day hospice staff need to facilitate the communication between patient and family if it has broken down. Often getting away to the day hospice a day or two each week allows patient and family to have different experiences to share with one another. If it can be a positive experience for the patient, the carer is freed from the guilt of enjoying 'time off' from caring.

There are many who have tried to enlighten us towards a meaning behind the suffering that terminally ill patients and their families inevitably go through even in the absence of distressing symptoms.[9, 10] Byock in addressing this subject[11] speaks about listening for what has meaning and, on occasions, invites patients to look at the events of their illness as the middle portion of a poignant novel:

> ... If we know the hero or heroine could not survive, what would be the best possible outcome of the story? Can you imagine or can we together imagine, perhaps a final two chapters that might leave the reader sad, but also feeling happy for the protagonist and with a sense of fullness or completion?

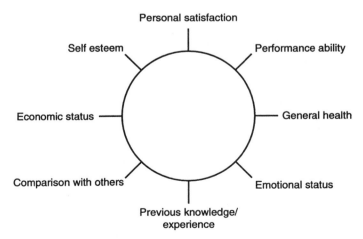

Quality of life

Personal satisfaction

Self esteem

Performance ability

Economic status

General health

Comparison with others

Emotional status

Previous knowledge/ experience

Fig. 2.1 Factors associated with quality of life (adapted from Patterson, 1975).[8]

Such an exercise can help refocus on what is important. It is not denying the inevitableness of death – that will always remain in the picture – but the focus is changed to the time that's left. Such work takes commitment, genuine compassion, and a willingness to invest the necessary emotional energy. This need not always be as intense as it sounds and can be genuinely satisfying. However, it often needs time, several months if possible. The day hospice has to become a place where the patient feels comfortable, and safe, in order to build up the rapport and trust necessary to do such work.

The rehabilitative team

The rehabilitative team will vary from place to place depending on resources and need. Such a team should consist of both professionals and skilled volunteers.

A full team can consist of a physiotherapist, chiropodist, art and music therapists, chaplains of all faiths, appliance fitter, doctor, speech therapist, volunteers, occupational therapist, diversional therapist, nurse specialists (stoma, continence, lymphoedema), social worker, dental hygienist, dietitians, home care community liaison, hairdresser, masseurs. Clearly, however, to have such a team all paid full time would be impossible. It may be quite sufficient to have just a nucleus of these skilled people and then be able to draw on the expertise of the chiropodist or the appliance fitter when the specific need arises. One cannot stress enough, however, the important position that the patient and the family play as members of the rehabilitation team.

To be able to acknowledge and identify patient self worth, self esteem, etc., team members clearly need to be aware of the affirmation of such qualities in their own lives.

Rehabilitation and re-adjustment

The potential of the day hospice in helping a patient to learn to live despite the prognosis of a terminal illness is enormous, but it takes tremendous insight and commitment. What is fundamental for a patient wanting to *live* in such a situation? This is difficult to answer; indeed there may not be just one answer. None the less, 'hope' is an underlying criterion for living and therefore must play its part, even in a terminal illness. But, how can a terminally ill patient 'hope'?

'Hope' in today's western civilisation tends to imply a positive outcome of good. However, this may not be so vital an interpretation. Travelbee (1971)[12] describes hope as 'a mental state characterised by the desire to gain an end or accomplish a goal combined with some degree of expectation that what is desired or sought is attainable'.

Herth (1990)[13] has identified seven 'hope fostering' strategies (Table 2.1) within the context of terminal illness. This piece of research interviewing 30 patients provides an important contribution to understanding the hoping process and how it may be used to enhance coping. It is important to emphasise that no-one can give hope to people – in Herth's language we can only foster hope.

These strategies can be further categorised into four sections which are most relevant as a means of rehabilitation in a day hospice situation: relationships, humour and reliving memories, inner strength, and goal setting.

Table 2.1 Key categories of hope fostering strategies[13]

Category level	Defining characteristics
Interpersonal/connectedness	Presence of meaningful, shared relationship(s) with another person(s)
Affirmation of worth	Having one's individuality accepted, honoured and acknowledged
Lightheartedness	Feeling of delight, joy or playfulness that is communicated verbally or non-verbally
Uplifting memories	Recalling positive moments
Personal attributes	Attributes of determination, courage and serenity
Spiritual base	Presence of active spiritual beliefs
Attainable aims	Directing efforts at some purpose

Relationships

As has already been hinted, many patients referred to a day hospice can be physically and emotionally isolated; either because of their disease or a pre-existing isolation exacerbated by the illness. The trauma of diagnosis, sometimes treatment, and a poor prognosis can either cement a family strongly together or can cause numerous defensive walls to be built around individuals. In the former instance the patient can often become smothered by good intentions and be prematurely ricocheted into a dependent invalid state, as everyone seeks to help. The latter situation can lead to a feeling of rejection and a difficulty in expressing feelings to one another.

Guilt about being ill is a common feature. Patients often feel a burden on people: the family, for being required to visit or to be put to more trouble than usual; the carers, for having to come and do for them things that normally they would have preferred to do for themselves if they were able. The guilt engenders a feeling of unconnectedness; it's important for these patients to feel important. In many respects it may be easier for team members to feel a kinship towards a 27-year-old patient terminally ill from carcinoma of the cervix. However, the challenge is the old bachelor, terminally ill, but with few friends and who has little conversation. Can we promote a shared relationship between him and the rest of the team?

The rediscovery that others are willing to invest in a relationship encourages self worth. Joining in cards, dominoes and other group games increases self confidence, as a patient successfully relates to others. The use of dining tables cements groups over the very normal social activity of eating. Given the difficulty caused by poor appetites which can cause friction at home with carers, it is important that meals are varied. There is no place for pre-served meals – food should be apportioned individually at the table to suit the differing appetites.

Humour and reliving memories

Humour in any situation is vital. However, one can get so caught up with the tragedy of illness that it can appear wrong to laugh and enjoy oneself in front of those less fortunate. This none the less is misleading. Many terminally ill patients need the rehabilitative team to bring them back into contact with what they have enjoyed in the past. Humour and laughter offer a release from the present. Visits from musicians, singers and actors bring patients in touch with areas of society from which they have become removed.

Some people are wary of reliving old memories with patients in case it reinforces what has passed. On the contrary, many want to be reminded of what has been good, and what has been achieved. Most people do have some good memories of fun and laughter times which can often relieve the boredom of the inactive lifestyle forced upon them through the weakness associated with terminal illness. Reminiscence work is an affirmation of the person who pre-existed the illness and of the person who exists now. Reliving past experiences can often reveal memories shared with contemporaries which renews happiness. It can also prove to be a spiritual journey that can put a patient and staff back in touch with the person of the past, before the illness clouded the image.

Inner strengths

There is no doubt that some people are naturally more hopeful than others. A positive nature in someone often endears people to them, and makes it easier for that person to foster hope. Victor Frankl's (1963)[9] work in his book *Man's search for meaning* exemplifies this ability of some to overcome deep hardship with an inner strength that helps them to find a reason, a purpose behind the suffering. Such determination or persistence in hope has appeared to be what keeps them going. Faith in a higher being or a spirituality often provides a sense of meaning that transcends human explanation.

Goal setting

Despite failing physical ability, small attainable aims help to give the sense that time is not just standing still waiting for the inevitable. Instead there is a moving forward in time which helps to nurture a degree of hope and usefulness. Even the basic everyday need of being able to eat a meal can be used to encourage a sense of achievement. To eat a small amount from a large helping is a negative experience but to clear a plate, however small the portion, is a positive achievement, which increases self esteem.

Such a philosophy of realistic hope is something that needs to be infused by the whole rehabilitative team. Most people who are terminally ill do realise the futility of continuing curative treatments but none the less feel abandoned when they are no longer regularly seen at the clinic. Being involved in a weekly or twice weekly visit to a day hospice not only prevents patients from feeling isolated, but helps to stop them from feeling that 'there's nothing more to be done'.

Uncertainty about the future inevitably brings with it a feeling of being out of control. Because so much of our life is about having choice and being in control, this uncertainty is very difficult to live with. Bringing back a degree of control and choice in areas not specifically related to the disease boosts self worth and confidence despite failing health.

John: a case study

The following case study has been a very encouraging example of how someone can readjust and find pleasure in the terminal phase of his life alongside what an established day hospice team can offer. With all the problems of low self esteem, lack of family support/cohesion because of alcohol abuse, and isolation, John was encouraged to start reassessing what he could and would like to do within the day hospice context. He found a non-judgemental atmosphere willing to meet him. In being able to explore things at his own pace, he integrated into a group setting, relearning what it meant to feel valued. Many of the aspects of rehabilitation discussed in this chapter are emulated in what John and his family achieved.

John was a 55-year-old man who had worked as a baker before his diagnosis of cancer. He presented to the day hospice having undergone a radical dissection of neck nodes for squamous cell carcinoma of unknown primary. This had been followed by some radiotherapy. He had a known dependency on alcohol and was troubled by a cough. John lived with his wife and three of their four children; the youngest, who was 14 years old, had no memory of a father who did not drink. The financial drain and embarrassment of John's alcoholic-induced behaviour had adversely affected the family relationships, to the point that just prior to his illness, the marriage was almost completely broken down. His wife, however, admitted that despite the alcohol dependency, John had never been late or lost a day's work, even though he started work each morning at 04.00.

On referral to the day hospice, five aims were established with the day hospice team:

- To reduce John's isolation; he had not been going out except to the corner shop.
- To explore and possibly help John with introspection and sadness; he had been tentatively labelled as suffering from a reactive depression.
- Assess and monitor the tumour's progress.
- Give his wife, the main carer, time for herself.
- Allay John's fears of the hospice; day hospice extended hospice care from his home to the actual hospice building.

It was with quite a lot of reluctance that John agreed to attend the day hospice after promptings by the hospice home care nurse visiting him at home. His most forceful bargaining point was that if he came along to the day hospice no-one was to challenge his alcoholism. On his first visit, John arrived bearing his own supply of beer and cider along with his drugs. His small slightly stooped frame was highlighted by a large dressing on the side of his neck. As with all new patients, the various activities and services of the day hospice were highlighted for him, leaving him to choose those with which he wanted to be involved. As he sat in a corner apparently only interested in his alcohol, staff and volunteers alike respected his decision. He gave every indication of low self worth and feelings of hopelessness.

Gradually, after regular attendance at the day hospice and observing the various group activities, John began to relate to other patients who came in on the same days. They too respected John's privacy regarding his alcohol; his behaviour did not offend, nor did it impinge on their enjoyment in the day hospice. After a number of visits a small group developed, sharing common symptoms and difficulties; they also began to reminisce about their lives. Slowly John joined in and began to talk about the man behind his illness and eventually beyond the alcohol. He was an accomplished cook and was soon taking interest in cooking demonstrations in the day hospice. As he had worked as a baker he was a fountain of knowledge and connoisseur of breads and cakes. A volunteer shared an interest in baking and encouraged John to talk about his wealth of information as well as occasionally taking him out to sample local bakeries. During one such visit, the restaurant chosen was the old site of a bakery where he had once worked.

In time, John was a regular popular winner of light hearted quizzes in the day hospice, and acknowledged by the group as a self-taught expert on Scottish history. After discovering that John was a keen reader of a local author, a visit from the author was arranged. Despite a deterioration in his physical condition, John was able to demonstrate his intimate knowledge of all the novels he had read. This enabled others to see that John was extremely well-read on topics that interested him. The achievement of the goal in meeting the author meant a great deal in the latter stages of John's illness.

During his time in the day hospice he developed a genuine interest in the other patients, often making new people feel relaxed. Initially, he attended the day hospice twice a week, but in response to his wife's increasing tiredness, he agreed to come three times a week. His wife had previously done the necessary dressings to his neck; now he allowed more help. As his tumour increased in size, the dressings required daily changes and the day hospice nurse liaised with the district nurse to offer consistent care. He also agreed to help with bathing following a fall in which he fractured his femur. Despite an excellent recovery, due to his own determination and commitment to exercises, he was less able to maintain his own care at home and relied more and more on the facilities at the day hospice.

John was always offered the chance to participate in various outings. He was embarrassed by his tumour with the need of large dressings, and always anxious that it be hidden under a scarf if he was in a public place so as not to offend others. During what was to be the last month of his life, John accompanied others from the day hospice on a visit into the countryside. On a beautiful spring day, he sat slightly to one side of the group and spoke of his happiness in just 'being there'. A real rehabilitative step for the man who had arrived at the day hospice as sad, introspective and hopeless.

He was encouraged to maintain control in as many areas as possible, highlighted by his directions to the hairdresser to keep the long hair of his youth. As his time at the day hospice increased he spent more and more time discussing his 'forthcoming death', its meaning for the family and in particular his plans for his own funeral. He made very precise detailed requests, including the use of particular pieces of music. The fact that the patients knew that the family fulfilled these, gave them satisfaction for John and hope for the fulfilment of their own wishes. John became an important member of the group.

When he was admitted to the hospice for in-patient care the remainder of his group visited him when he was unable to get up to the day hospice himself. Members of the group expressed their thankfulness at being able to say 'goodbye'. After his death, his friends continued to talk affectionately about the time he had spent with them. A true example of the change from the isolated man first admitted to the day hospice to someone who had reminisced about his livelihood as a baker, who had spoken about his happiness at just 'being' in the countryside, to a man of courage able to make a recovery after fracturing his femur in the terminal phase of his illness and then to speak openly about death and organise his own funeral.

In conclusion, the day hospice had provided a safe environment in which John was able to explore his life, and rediscover his value and self esteem. Those who understood his medical condition and yet offered a non-judgemental attitude affirmed his worth as a person. Enjoying activities and achieving goals, led to an improvement in his psychological condition, giving him hope in terms of quality of life. John's time in the day hospice relieved symptoms as they developed and eased his fears of hospice care, helping him to live life in the fullest way possible until his death as an in-patient.

His family were able to see the rehabilitation in John and in the main were able to see the man beyond the illness and alcohol. They valued him enough to fulfil to the letter his requests for his funeral arrangements and prior to that had given him the chance to discuss these freely. Finally, the response to the request to base this case study on John's experience was one of joy, in the assurance that John would have been pleased and their own genuine pleasure that he had been suggested. John's destination of his journey through the terminal phase of cancer was never in doubt, but he moved from third class travel to first class travel as he took advantage of the 'rehabilitation' offered.

Conclusion

The progressive illness which brings with it diminishing function in terminal illness is a challenge of rehabilitation that is far greater and yet more subtle than other rehabilitation units or day care. To take the train analogy a little further – perhaps it is the difference between the terminally ill patient being the passenger in a car and the actual driver of the car. Being a passenger one is taken here and there. However, being a driver of the car gives one the freedom to choose where to go and when to stop. A terminal illness doesn't need to be a passive acceptance of being told what to do because of the inevitable. Our responsibility as health workers in a day hospice is to enable people attending the centre to experience a feeling of importance and self-worth in their lives. The day hospice team becomes the co-driver; enabling the patient, 'the driver', to make choices about what they would like or like not to do. The rehabilitation team within a day hospice needs to be 'alive', 'alert' to the journey that the patient is on.

References

1. Nicholson W. *Shadowlands*. London: Samuel French, 1990.
2. Macleod PJ. The problem of rehabilitation. In: *Rehabilitation – the report of the Medical Advisory Committee (Scotland)*. Edinburgh: HMSO, 1946.
3. Dietz JH. Rehabilitation of the cancer patient. *Med Clin North Am* 1969; **53**: 3.
4. Dietz JH. *Rehabilitation in oncology*. New York: John Wiley, 1981.
5. Hockley, J. Rehabilitation in palliative care – are we asking the impossible? *Palliative Med* 1993; **7 (suppl. 1)**: 9–15.
6. Holmes S, Dickerson J. The quality of life: design and evaluation of a self-assessment instrument for use with cancer patients. *Int J Nursing Studies* 1987; **1**: 15–24.
7. Buckman R. *I don't know what to say*. London: Macmillan Papermac, 1988.
8. Patterson W. The quality of survival in response to treatment. *J Am Med Assoc* 1995; **233**: 280–1.
9. Frankl VE. *Man's search for meaning*. Boston: Beacon Press, 1963.
10. Cassel E. The nature of suffering: physical, psychological, social and spiritual aspects. In: Stark P., McGovern J., eds. *The hidden dimension of illness: human suffering*. New York: National League for Nursing Press, 1992.
11. Bycock, I. When suffering persists. *J Palliative Care* 1994; **2**: 8–13.
12. Travelbee J. Concept: Hope. In: *Interpersonal aspects of nursing*, 2nd edn. Philadelphia: Davis Publishing Company, 1971.
13. Herth K. Fostering hope in terminally-ill people. *J advanced nursing* 1990; **15**: 1250–9.

3

The National Health Service and Community Care Act 1990

Shirley Parnis

Over the last few years there have been major changes in the way health and social care is being delivered within the community in Great Britain. The familiar role of the home help providing assistance with shopping, laundry and cleaning, is being replaced by care assistants and nursing auxiliaries with the emphasis on personal care rather than on domestic help in the home. The introduction of the National Health Service and Community Care Act, 1990, which became fully operational in April, 1993, implemented the recommendations made by Sir Roy Griffiths in his paper *Caring for people*.[1] His review of community care services highlighted the regional variations in the provision of services, the spiralling costs of care, and most importantly, that insufficient attention was paid to 'service users' and carers' preferences',[2] namely, what the client/patient and their families wanted. This review resulted in local authority Social Services Departments becoming the lead agency for social care, with a responsibility for ensuring adequate provision of care in the community 'in this decade and beyond'.[1] Consequently, unlimited Government funds were directed away from the Department of Social Security who previously paid for nursing and residential placements when insufficient care and support had been available in the community, with limited funds now allocated to local authorities to implement care in the community.

Therefore the aim of the NHS and Community Care Act, 1990, is to give people greater independence and choice with the opportunity to live and be cared for wherever possible in their own homes, with sufficient support for this to be viable. The Act, for the first time, formally recognised the importance of the carers' role in looking after sick or disabled relatives, neighbours or friends as often they had been the main or only carer and had received inadequate community support. Existing legislation relating to service provision for the sick and disabled, as well as the elderly and the mentally ill, is covered by several Acts of Parliament, in addition to various directives issued by the Secretary of State. Together they provide a complex legal framework with the NHS and Community Care Act, 1990, being the most recent legislation. In this Act the Government has set out six key objectives which attempt to bring about a change of attitude and approach in the provision of social care, and these can be summarised as follows:

- to promote the development of domiciliary day and respite services to enable people to live in their own homes wherever feasible and sensible;
- to ensure that service providers make practical support for carers a high priority;

- to make an assessment of need and good care management the cornerstone of high quality care;
- to promote the development of a flourishing independent sector alongside good quality public services;
- to clarify the responsibilities of agencies and to make it easier to hold them to account for their performance;
- to secure better value for taxpayers' money by introducing a new structure for social care.[3]

In addition the NHS and Community Care Act, 1990, has encouraged local authorities to separate the roles of purchase and provision of services, with an assessment for care becoming 'needs led' rather than 'services led' which had generally been the practice pre-April 1993. This major change in policy is aimed at ensuring that as well as offering more individual choice, the client and their carers are consulted about the type of services required, and that these services meet the identified 'needs', via a needs-led assessment. Although the assessment should focus on the difficulties for which individuals are seeking assistance, Government guidance given to local authorities prior to the Act's full implementation in April 1993, stated that:

> it should also take into account all of the circumstances relevant to those individuals, such as, their capacities and incapacities; their preferences and aspirations; their living situation and the support available from friends, and any other source of help. This information provides the context for subsequent decisions about what services (if any) will be provided.[4]

Therefore the NHS and Community Care Act, 1990, attempts to ensure that the emphasis of community care is focused on enabling people to remain in their own homes by the promotion and provision of a high standard of health, local authority and independent sector community care. This includes domiciliary care, day care and respite care in order to prevent unnecessary admissions to hospitals, nursing homes or residential establishments if this is not the assessed need or preferred choice. An increasing range of palliative care services, such as hospice care which includes pain/symptom control and respite admissions, palliative day care, hospital at home, Macmillan nurses and Marie Curie nursing combined with local authority community care, can enable patients with life-threatening illnesses to be cared for in their own homes. These services recognise the individual's needs and preferences, and are in accord with the intentions of the Act. They also achieve the goal of allowing families and their network of carers to be involved in the care of a patient with the added confidence that they are supported by both the primary health care team, such as the general practitioner and district nurses, in addition to the multi-disciplinary palliative care team which includes both professionals and volunteers, providing a range of medical, emotional and practical support. Many of these professionals would be asked to contribute to the needs-led assessment and care planning process.

Although the Act requires that local authority Social Services Departments are the lead agency for assessing care, in many areas of the country a needs-led assessment may be carried out by a number of different health or social services professionals. Whichever accredited professional undertakes to carry out a needs-led assessment they will be known as the 'assessor', 'care coordinator' or 'care manager' as the title varies regionally. The needs-led assessment can be undertaken in a variety of settings, for example, at home, in a day care setting or even in hospital, and should be carried out in consultation with the patient, their carers and the other professionals involved in their treatment or care. The assessment is aimed at identifying the client/patient's 'needs' in areas such as, personal care, mobility, household tasks, as well as physical and mental health issues, including any housing or financial needs. For example, in carrying out an assessment of 'mobility needs' this would include an assessment of any difficulties in: walking, transferring from a bed to a chair or to a toilet/commode, or in managing stairs. Once the assessment is completed the assessor would consider whether or not these difficulties could be overcome in the home, with the provision of aides, adaptations or personal help. In a complex assessment, an occupational therapist, or other professionals, may be asked to contribute to the assessment process.

Once the care needs have been identified and recorded, the assessor will draw up an appropriate care plan which sets out in detail how each specific 'need' will be met, by whom, when, where, how often, at what time, etc. A copy of the assessment and written notification of any 'needs' which cannot be met should also be supplied in addition to a copy of the care plan. Local authorities are allowed to make a charge for the services they commission or provide and they can determine their own charging policy. This is currently rather a contentious issue as the charge can range from a fixed fee to a scale rate depending on the number of hours of care provided by, or commissioned from, an independent agency on behalf of the Social Services Department. However, the care plan should clearly indicate the full cost of the care package and what contribution the service user is expected to pay. Payment of benefits such as the care component of the Disability Living Allowance (under pension age) and Attendance Allowance, are intended to help with the cost of care needs.

In a palliative care setting most care plans will indicate that a combination of health and social care is required, especially when there are considerable health issues which may fluctuate or change quickly. In these situations it is usually appropriate to review the assessment and care plan frequently to reflect the changes in the identified 'needs'. The shifting balance of responsibility for health and social provision in the community has led to some confusion about exactly who is responsible for the purchase and provision of some services, and how the costs of these will be met. For example, is an assessed 'need' for help with a bath or personal care a health or a social need, and which provider should meet this care need? This is currently a subject of controversy as the outcome of this decision will influence whether or not a charge for the service will be required from the service user. The introduction of the NHS and Community Care Act, 1990, has had enormous financial implications for local authorities and Social Services Departments who have had to put in place a new infrastructure to implement the Act. Obviously differences in how Health and Social Services Departments are structured and administered has, in some areas of the country, resulted in difficulties in determining who is, or should be, the purchaser and provider of services.

However, in order to meet the criteria outlined in the NHS and Community Care Act, 1990, both Health and Social Service providers were required to establish agreed protocols of how services will be commissioned and provided, and in many areas this has resulted in closer working relationships between the two. Details of what services are available, who is the provider, how services are accessed and delivered, have all had to be clarified in a local 'Community Care Plan' prior to the final implementation of the Act in April 1993. Local plans continue to vary regionally, but should be available for public inspection which is an attempt to ensure that service providers become more accountable. The NHS and Community Care Act, 1990, also required local authorities to introduce a complaints procedure in order that any query or disagreement about the assessment process, the allocation and any shortfalls of services, or any other complaint could be appropriately dealt with. Since the introduction of the Act there has been a considerable increase in the amount of administration necessary in undertaking a needs-led assessment and coordinating a care plan which can lead to delays in completing assessments or in providing services in some regions. Increased public expectations and greater demand for services, together with an ageing population and a reduction in residential provision, has resulted in many local authorities struggling to meet the demands required by the Act within the limited funds available to them.

However, for community care to offer genuine care options and client choice, continued collaboration and effective communication remains essential between the providers of health and social care. An increasing trend towards the commissioning of joint health and social provision of services is an attempt at providing a 'seamless' service. This also has the advantage of avoiding some of the current difficulties in determining who should be the purchaser and service provider when there are local disagreements, or an overlap of health and social care needs. Certainly as family networks have become smaller and socially more isolated in Britain, there has been a growing awareness and acceptance that for clients/patients to be cared for, and supported in the community, the responsibility for this has to be shared between the individual and the State. The initial findings of some research carried out within the first year of the NHS and Community Care Act's full implementation, when examining emerging themes, confirmed that the first impressions of care in the community were favourable: 'there was a broadly based commitment to the concept of community care' and that the 'energy which had been focused on plans, systems and structures was beginning to be redirected into independent living opportunities and community based services'.[5] It was anticipated by Sir Roy Griffiths that the full implications of the Act would not be effective immediately as both the National Health Service administration and local authority Social Services Departments would need a reasonable period of time to assess, plan and organise the resources required to meet local care needs. Therefore decisions about the purchasing of services, their delivery, resource and cost implications, etc., are still areas which need to be clarified and resolved.

Although this paper has focused on the introduction of a recent piece of British legislation, the aims and intentions of the Act, in attempting to promote care in the community in Britain, may be of some value to other countries when planning or reviewing their own community-based palliative care services. This may apply in particular to those professionals and volunteers who are working in this field in countries where the extended family network has largely disappeared. This is especially relevant where there is a growing need for health and social care agencies to become involved in, and to organise, appropriate palliative care provision. However in Britain, a Government commitment to adequate funding of care in the community is desperately needed if the intentions behind the implementation of the NHS and Community Care Act, 1990 are to be achieved. In addition, for community care to be effective it is also essential that everyone involved works together with shared aims and goals, if they are to offer clients/patients with life-threatening illnesses, or any other assessed need or disability, the opportunity to maximise their quality of life and to realise their full potential. In order to achieve this, first both the patient and their carers need to be consulted and to participate fully in the assessment and care planning processes; and second, patients should be given 'real' care choices that will empower them and promote a greater level of control, independence and dignity in being cared for in the community.

The NHS and Community Care Act, 1990, adequately funded and implemented should, over the next decade, help to achieve this in Great Britain.

References

1. Secretaries for Health, Social Security, Wales and Scotland. *Caring for people: community care in the next decade and beyond.* London: HMSO, 1989.
2. Griffiths R. *Community care: agenda for action.* London: HMSO, 1988.
3. Parnis SE. The Community Care Act . . . and you. *Palliative Care Services J* 1993; 2: 12.
4. Chief Inspector, Social Services Inspectorate. *Implementing caring for people: assessment.* C1(92)34, 1990.
5. Department of Health. *Implementing caring for people – impressions of the first year.* London: DOH, 1994.

4

Palliative care in motor neurone disease

Ann Stead and Gavin Jenkins

Introduction

Amyotrophic lateral sclerosis/motor neurone disease (MND) is a progressive disease, the course of which from diagnosis to death can be infinitely variable. For the majority the prognosis is a few years at best of relentless progression of disabilities. The life of the person with MND, and equally of their care givers, is one of constant readjustment to a changing level of ability as the function of one group of muscles after another is lost.

To date there is no known cure for MND and yet this does not mean that the situation is hopeless, as psychological, physical and/or pharmacological methods of some kind are available to help to alleviate symptoms and to compensate for, or overcome, at least in part, disability. Palliative care in the context of this chapter refers not only to the management of the later stages of the disease, as is often traditionally thought, but to the whole process of care in a condition where there is no cure.

Description

Motor neurone disease (MND) is so called because it is characterised by a selective degeneration of the motor neurones involving both the corticospinal pathways and those which originate in the motor nuclei of the brainstem and the anterior horn cells of the spinal cord. The three cranial nerves which control the movement of the eyes, and the lower sacral segments of the spinal cord are spared (not applicable to very advanced stages of MND especially when artificial ventilation is being used). The autonomic nervous system and the sensory nerves are not affected. Intellect and memory remain intact throughout in the vast majority of cases.

Epidemiology

MND occurs, with a fairly uniform distribution, in all countries of the world. It has a prevalence thought to be between eight to ten per 100 000 and an incidence of approximately 1 per 50 000 per year. It is predominantly a disease of later middle life with an average age of onset of 56 years. Men are more often affected in a ratio of about two to one and 5 to 10 per cent of cases are familial. There are also some intriguing pockets of the disease in the world where very high incidents of disorders that are either very similar or identical to MND have been found, the most well known of these being the island of Guam.

Progression

Onset is insidious, with the initial stages, speed and pattern of progression of the disease varying widely between individuals. Common first signs are stumbling, weakened grip, cramps or a hoarse voice, progressing to loss of function of limbs and weakness and wasting of muscles of the trunk and neck, and this can lead to total dependence.

Types of presentation

There are three forms of MND:

Amyotrophic lateral sclerosis (ALS)

This is the most common form of MND involving both upper and lower motor neurones characterised by muscle weakness, spasticity, hyperactive reflexes and emotional lability. Age of onset is usually over 55 years and the average survival from diagnosis is 3–4 years.[1]

Progressive muscular atrophy (PMA)

PMA is a predominantly lower motor neurone degeneration causing muscle wasting and weakness with loss of weight and fasciculation (muscle twitching). In this case the age of onset is usually under 50 years with male predominance and with the majority of people surviving beyond 5 years from diagnosis.[1]

Progressive bulbar palsy (PBP)

This is paralysis of the bulbar muscles by a lower motor neurone lesion of the cranial nerves controlling speech and swallowing. Speech is hypernasal and slurred and deteriorates to a point of total loss of functional speech. Swallowing difficulties cause choking on food and drink; pooling of saliva and dribbling. Many people remain ambulant to the end but muscles in the upper limbs and shoulder girdle may become progressively weaker. PBP occurs mostly in older people, is slightly more common in women and survival from onset of symptoms is usually between 6 months and 3 years.[1]

It is important to stress that MND affects each individual very differently in respect of symptoms in the initial stages, the rate of progression of the disease and survival time after the diagnosis and for many people death intervenes before they experience all possible symptoms.

Providing support services

The provision of palliative care for MND is a relatively new concept. Most neurological conditions causing physical disability, e.g. multiple sclerosis, progress at a much slower rate and are perceived to be 'disabilities' as opposed to illnesses. MND on the other hand can have a speed of progression more akin to conditions such as cancers and certainly requires a similar mobilisation of resources to help. Pain, however, is not a major feature of MND. It certainly exists, particularly in relation to immobility, but its physiological similarities with cancer are limited. The palliative care and hospice movements are now beginning to realise that they have a great deal to offer people with MND; unfortunately, however, the reality is that many people are passed from agency to agency and few find adequate support.

It is important that perception of 'illness' and 'disability' are understood as this will affect the attitudes of the person with MND and the type of support they choose. One person may feel more comfortable in a day centre for the physically disabled, whilst another may prefer a more reflective environment such as a hospice. The vast majority of people prefer to be cared for and die at home in which case the environment may require adaptation to cope with increasing physical limitations. Similarly environmental factors will need to be considered if care is offered away from home and basic requirements such as a reclining seat, adequate space for a wheelchair, hoists and alarm call systems will be necessary for most people, particularly in the later stages.

There are many differing approaches to the management of MND; specialist neurological or disability teams, or palliative care teams may be available but in many instances it's a lone physician, therapist or nurse struggling to provide whatever help is available. There is no ideal model that meets the needs of everyone with MND as each person will require a different approach depending upon their personality and lifestyle. There are, however, three guiding principles which must underpin every care package: client centredness; continuity and comprehensiveness. These principles must span the health and social care divide.

The first is that services must be client centred. Personal ambitions and desires about what to do with whatever life remains must be the foundation of a service. Treatment regimes, diagnostic and support services must not form the focus of provision; these are secondary aspects which should support primary aims relating to quality of life. To those familiar with the term client- or person–centredness it may seem unnecessary to mention this; however, many services still operate on a very medical model which sees the diagnosis first and the person second. All health care professionals should try to evaluate their current practice from the point of view of the person with MND and ask is it offering what the individual needs? An example of this is a gentleman who visited the Mary Marlborough Centre in Oxford, UK, and was assessed by the then medically orientated inter-disciplinary team which had identified a number of problems ranging from transfer techniques to independent feeding; when asked what his main priority was, the 'patient' answered 'to be able to release my homing pigeons for the last time myself!'. He had little or no interest in feeding himself or being able to stand to transfer. Reappraising their narrow vision, the team then set to work designing a release mechanism for his pigeon basket for the man to use with his limited grip and taught his carers about feeding and transfers. The centre has since completely restructured itself and adopted a much more client–centred approach.

The second major guiding principle is continuity; once a service is involved it must maintain an ongoing commitment. Continuity is critical where rapid change occurs and where speech will become increasingly impaired. Getting to know the person and their family well before crises occur smoothes the path for all concerned and helps everyone to know the person's wishes for future management. Advance directives and living wills are all part of this philosophy. Key workers are vital, yet this role is emotionally draining so adequate supervision and sharing of this load is important.

As new problems arise people will be referred to specialist services for all manner of help. They are likely to be assessed and reassessed, telling their story endlessly. Key workers who know the person well can smooth out these bureaucratic anomalies and provide the necessary information in advance. This is particularly important in the later stages of the diseases where speech may be impaired. Anticipating needs early gives time to build trust, to adjust the care programme and avoids distress. Introducing new carers in a time of crisis can be most distressing for all concerned.

The key worker will need to assess and reassess the situation on a regular basis, probably monthly. They must see the problems first hand which means in the person's home. In this way plans can be made and problems anticipated. When specialist equipment is needed there is no time for waiting lists or Social Services committees to determine priorities. Equipment provided too early is likely to be rejected, so items should be on stand-by or money should have been reserved for when the time is right. It should be remembered, however, that equipment does have its limitations.

There can be a tendency to assume that technology can improve upon human function. Good as it is, synthesised speech fails to hold any of the nuances of human wit or candour. It is a poor replacement for human speech and people should be given truthful information about the usefulness of equipment. Funding is often problematic in conditions such as MND that span the health and social divide; therefore before any equipment is suggested, thought should be given to payment and the realistic possibility of provision. Also the design of some equipment can be off-putting. Hoists are big and clumsy and can dominate a room. Care must also be used when introducing equipment. If introduced sensitively it is likely to be successful, if not its rejection will increase the carer's work load.

The final guiding principle is that the service should be comprehensive. For people who have major mobility and postural impairments, it is unreasonable to ask them to visit centre after centre when travel is difficult and they become rapidly fatigued. Apart from the inefficiency of repeated assessment and history taking, solutions to problems should form an integrated package of care. Advice on seating, computers, communication and environmental systems, finance, nutrition and medication should all be available under one roof, preferably on the same day by a team experienced in the management of MND. Solving one problem without due regard to other aspects of management is time wasting and counter-productive. If it is not possible to find a service that offers this type of team work in one place, the key worker should try to organise the various key players to come to the person's home or work place and work together. Health and social service systems are notoriously slow and people with MND do not have time for statutory services to mobilise into action. It is not uncommon with someone with MND to be provided with a head support which provides comfort for rest and relaxation, but is ineffective when using a communication aid or a wheelchair control. Every aspect of movement or function will impact upon another and the person's needs and the service's ability to respond must be viewed in totality to have any hope of being effective. The case management then needs to be reviewed regularly.

The number of agencies with which a person with MND will become involved is likely to be huge. Health and social services will be the key players but housing, benefits and information agencies may also become involved. Of course, people have their own networks of support such as professional or social clubs, churches, disability groups, friends and neighbours. The main health care professionals involved throughout the course of the disease will be general practitioners, neurologists, occupational therapists, physiotherapists, nurses, speech and language therapists and dieticians. Just who from this vast array the person with MND chooses to be their key worker doesn't matter and it may differ as circumstances change. No single profession has all the answers. What matters is that whoever is the key worker has a sense of what should be done, how to anticipate problems and who to contact for help and when. Professional jealousies and pettiness have no place in this scenario and the individual with MND should be free to choose their key worker in the knowledge that he or she will be respected by all the others involved and that they will receive the necessary support they require as time passes.

Management

Working with a person with MND stretches the skills of the professional to the full because of the emotional demands of a life-threatening disease, and because of the rapid progression of the disease often meaning that his or her functional ability will alter from week to week, or even day to day. Throughout this, individuals will retain an alert and active mind, even when speech and movement are lost to them. Everything possible should be done to allow them to make their views and needs known, allowing them to continue to control their life and the decisions that affect them.

Yet within this the problems that they will face are no different from problems faced by people with other neurological conditions. Why then is the management of MND such a challenge and what skills are needed when faced with it?

In short, the greatest challenges that must be overcome are firstly the immense speed with which this condition can progress, stretching services to the limit, and secondly professional prejudices and limitations. There appears to be a mystique to the label of MND that renders some health professionals unable to respond and perhaps in some way fearful. Whilst this fear is, in some instances, understandable it is important to remember that for many health professionals their training and working life is dedicated to problem-solving and the problems associated with MND have probably been seen before under a different label.

More than anything else the greatest service one can do for people with MND is to listen to them and act on what they say. One must remember that they are living with this problem and very often have formulated ideas to help themselves; they need no more than a facilitator to allow these ideas to come into being.

The key is to concentrate on enabling the person to achieve more and to focus efforts on quality of life. Advances in technology are offering tremendous opportunities to enhance the quality of life experienced by an individual with a severe disability, more so than ever before, and surely the role of the health professionals is to harness the power of this revolution to benefit their client.

What therefore are the needs of the person with MND? What are the needs of any person? There is no simple answer to these questions; however, by breaking down the elements of human function into key groupings, a framework emerges that allows the identification of the skills needed to minimise these effects.

The elements of human function affected by MND are likely to be:

Respiration

The feeling of not being able to take in enough air is common. Within the condition the respiratory muscles may become weaker and so lead to dyspnoea, and a survey showed evidence of this in 60 per cent of cases.[2] Careful positioning and a confident calm approach by people around can help. Dyspnoea may be eased by sitting reclined; tobacco smoke and excessive central heating should be avoided.

Coughing and choking are defence mechanisms to prevent the aspiration of liquids and solids into the lungs. Persistent choking or ineffective coughing calls for techniques to improve comfort, alleviate distress and ensure aspiration does not worsen.

Simple portable suction machines can be used to remove oral secretions and if required with proper instruction this can be used within the home environment. The pooling of saliva in the pharynx is distressing and uncomfortable and the use of a suction machine can improve the comfort and dignity of the person. Medication can also assist in the alleviation of excess salivation and medical advice should be sought.[3] Radiotherapy of the salivary glands has also been shown to provide some temporary relief.

The use of ventilators to extend life is still not common within the UK, but is increasingly used within countries such as the USA. There is a complex interweaving of medical, legal and ethical issues within this small and controversial area, as well as many practical problems that need to be overcome; however, the option of choosing this method of intervention is a very real one and the technology is available to allow this to happen. It is, however, a decision that needs to be discussed very carefully, prior to the crisis point and with full knowledge of the consequences and due to its complexity is beyond the scope of this passage.

Sleeping, a basic human function, may be disturbed in a person who is:

• unable to change position;
• unable to expend adequate energy during the day to warrant sleep;
• fearful or insecure.

Attention to detail, careful positioning, pressure-relieving mattresses, supportive cushions, mild sedation and an appropriate alarm call system may all assist and increase confidence in the individual, allowing them and their spouse/carer to sleep adequately.

Ingestion and digestion

There are several reasons why the person with MND may complain of difficulty in swallowing food or liquid. It is important for the speech and language therapist to establish accurately what level of difficulty is occurring; endoscopic and radiological investigations can be useful to do this. Common problems may include chewing or forming a bolus and propulsion of the bolus to the back of the mouth as a precursor to swallowing.

Swallowing difficulties in the early stages may be helped by a full explanation to the person of the normal swallowing processes. Changes in diet can greatly influence management of this problem – smooth but firm food with an even texture which can form a good bolus is the first step. Frequently liquids are more difficult than solids. At later stages semi-solid food may be tolerated. Crumbly foods should be avoided as it is difficult for the tongue to form a bolus. A dietician is an essential member of the team in preparing detailed and personal diet sheets.

Dysphagia may also be improved by replacing the automatic nature of a swallow with a more purposeful deliberate plan, offering the person greater control and confidence. Another important consideration is the environment as people may be aware that they are eating slowly, anxious about choking or embarrassed about the situation. A place where the person can relax and be comfortable is essential, as is eating smaller meals more often to reduce fatigue.[4]

Again these are only a few key ideas for consideration and the skills of a speech and language therapist and dietician are essential in the management of dysphagia. The advice and techniques needed will change during the course of the condition and the person will need to be monitored on a regular basis to control this symptom effectively.

When feeding becomes so laborious that it is no longer pleasurable and the person is becoming exhausted and depressed by the effort, consideration can be given to the use of alternative feeding such as gastrostomy. These simple procedures can overcome the burden of feeding and the constant struggle to obtain adequate nutrients and calories to maintain a healthy intake. It should be seen, and presented, as a positive step as it does not necessarily indicate the cessation of all oral intake but can allow the person to eat a quality diet, of the foodstuffs they enjoy, without the ordeal of quantity.

Movement

Experiencing difficulty or an inability to change one's position, for example to walk, sit, stand, turn; being unable to communicate through body language or to achieve comfort and relieve pain by a change of posture or to manipulate objects and interact with one's immediate environment are some of the consequences of loss of movement.

The person with MND is robbed of these abilities but, by modifying or assisting function with specialised equipment or replacing the function with an acceptable alternative, a person's life can be enhanced many times over.

The timing of the introduction of walking sticks and wheelchairs is important, as is the attitude of the prescriber. Introduced too early they can frighten and depress the person, too late means missed opportunities. They should be introduced as a means of achieving independence and choices and not as a response to their disability; a positive attitude from the prescriber is essential if a piece of equipment is to be welcomed.

The skills required to maintain movement are those of occupational therapy and physiotherapy in partnership with orthotics, bioengineering, electronic engineering and mechanical engineering to name but a small selection. The ability to move is fundamental to having purpose in one's life and maintaining self esteem. Without movement the person loses the ability to effect choices and decisions about life. Without the extensive range of technical equipment to compensate for the relentless weakening and erosion of physical abilities, the person with MND can become rapidly dependent upon others.[3]

Communication

Seventy-five per cent of people with MND experience difficulties with speech,[2] varying from slight slurring to total loss. The ability to communicate is such a fundamental need and all persons with any degree of dysarthria should be under the care of a speech and language therapist. An early referral system needs therefore to be established so that the person with MND has the opportunity for advice and speech conservation. Often people are not referred until their speech is totally unintelligible, whereas ideally if the person got to know their therapist before losing the ability to express themselves fully they could explain their own needs themselves.

The management of dysarthria comprises three general areas:

1. Explanation and description of the vocal tract; most people have no idea how they speak and providing them with information about the speech mechanism gives them something tangible to work on.
2. Speech conservation; this is appropriate when the person is not making the best use of the damaged system. The person could perhaps be offered a short course to learn how to improve their intelligibility. They need to learn to identify the abnormal features and monitor closely their speech as they attempt to modify production. At all times the emphasis must be on making the best use of the damaged mechanism of speech.
3. Strategies to improve communication; this area needs to be considered with both the person with MND and their carer, and the following points are worth discussing:

   • environment of communication
   • awareness of stress and fatigue on both the speaker's and listener's part
   • ensure all aids are used appropriately
   • encourage active communication at all times, do not speak for the person
   • be honest about difficulties in understanding what the person is saying and allow time for them to communicate fully.[4]

For many people with MND alternative and augmentative communication systems (AAC) become necessary as the disease progresses. The problem for the therapist is when to introduce the idea of an aid. Acceptance will usually be easier for the person if an aid can be introduced gradually while they are still using verbal communication. It may be suggested, for example, that the aid be used for specific situations where speech is more difficult. In this way the introduction of the aid does not signal a total loss of function.

Choice of the most appropriate aid is dependent upon a number of factors including the person's needs, be they either at home, work or socially; the environment in which it will be used; the person's physical abilities to operate the aid and their motivation.

As the person with MND experiences increasing difficulties, a combination of AAC systems will probably become necessary, with more complex electronic aids becoming essential.

A thorough assessment for the most suitable aid to fit individual needs and abilities is essential and with the rapid advances and developments in this area the advice of a centre specialising in AAC becomes imperative

Psychological aspects of MND

The relentless progression of MND, which may continue over an unknown number of months or years, is characterised by increasing physical dependence on others. This profound change inevitably takes its emotional toll on everyone who comes into contact with it. An overwhelming array of health care professionals and differing agencies will become involved in trying to support people through the uncharted journey.

For the person with MND each day can bring new losses. There is an unspoken expectation in society that even if a cure is unavailable, more should be done to alleviate the devastation MND brings in its wake. This is perhaps due to the speed of deterioration that often leaves little time for adjustment and acceptance. All of these factors can lead to feelings of hopelessness. However, there is a great deal that can be done to support people with MND and their families, and a positive and systematic approach to each problem as it arises is the most effective means of providing assistance.

Individual people react differently to the realisation that they have been diagnosed with MND. The degree of sensitivity in the way the diagnosis has been given will vary enormously. The ideal is that the person should be able to choose who is with them at the time this information is given and that they are offered an identified person to contact for ongoing support and information. Sadly, this does not always occur. Age, culture, personality and responsibilities will all affect how people react, but honesty and accurate information are the only means available which truly enable people to develop their own coping strategies, whatever they may be.

One of the cruellest manifestations of MND is that at a time when the most intimate fears and desires need to be shared as death approaches, the critical means of this expression – speech – is denied. It can be agonising for all concerned to witness the inadequacies of an inanimate communication aid being used to describe a person's last wishes. Painful though it is, people should be encouraged to talk about personal ambitions and critical issues whilst time allows and not leave things until it is too late. Common fears are about choking and how death will finally come. The Motor Neurone Disease Association in the UK have provided an information pack called the 'Breathing Space Kit' which includes small amounts of rapid action anxiolytics and pain relief for any acute medical emergencies that might induce panic at home. The medication is agreed with the general practitioner and is kept safely in the person's home should it be required in an emergency. Medico-legal issues in individual countries may make such initiatives impractical. However, the 'Breathing Space Kit' has proved to be of great value where it is in use.

Not surprisingly, depression is a common feature in MND. Occasionally this needs specialist treatment and it is important to recognise when any depressive phase becomes pathological. Depression is a natural reaction to coping with a deteriorating condition, as are all the features of a grief reaction such as anger and denial; with help and support these can be worked through. Occasionally, however, these reactions overwhelm people and specialist intervention may be necessary. This usually takes the form of counselling and/or medication and the general practitioner will make the necessary referrals.

It is particularly important to consider the psychological well-being of the family. For those who have adopted new roles, their position in the family may have changed from spouse and lover to that of carer. An active sex life may have diminished without discussion as the condition progresses and the care needs dominate. Carers should have access to an understanding and confidential listening ear for this and other issues. The needs of the carers are often overlooked when in fact their support mechanism may need to go on for much longer than the lifespan of the person with MND and their fears about the future will be very real and pressing. Offering support to the carer will make them feel more confident about their role and more able to cope. Contact with the Motor Neurone Disease Association should be made early. They provide excellent support through information counselling and advice through an international network and are able to grade the information in a way that is appropriate to the person's level of acceptance.

Tensions and stresses will emerge along the path as deterioration occurs and as landmarks are reached such as retiring from work, having to stop driving, using a wheelchair. Children often find conflict with their own demands for attention and care and feel guilty. Encouraging communication through open discussion with all the family at a level of understanding appropriate to the children's age is the best way of dealing with this.

One important aspect of MND is that although the physical disabilities are immense the intellect remains unaffected for the majority. This means that the person does not change. Support should therefore be directed at maintaining a quality of life through an acknowledgement that people should retain control in their lives and that personal wishes and ambitions are still fulfillable. Reduced time scales may change priorities and some things will become unattainable. However, the history books are filled with stunning examples of what the human spirit can achieve, and a diagnosis such as MND tends to focus minds on what is really important to people. Every effort should be made to realise this potential; practical problems can and should be overcome.

Quality of life

Living with a physical disability requires effective planning and the complexity of care packages can limit spontaneity. It will no longer be possible to catch a train for a long weekend away without detailed plans being drawn up. This does not mean, however, that people with physical disabilities should stop living. Holidays and leisure interests continue to be important. Indeed, quality time spent with family and interests in leisure pursuits will take priority.

The impact that new technology is having in society will mean that physical disability is no longer a bar to leading a full and exciting life. For the person with MND the path they must follow is one of advancing dependence and reliance upon others as they weaken to a point where they are unable to perform even the most basic task, – or is it? Technology means that electrical appliances can be controlled with a single switch, cars can be driven using a joy-stick, computers operated by speech, and even now trials are underway that will allow the operation of a wheelchair by just thinking of the direction of travel. It would seem that the benefits of technology are limitless. The challenge is to welcome this technology and direct it to meet the needs of people with physical disabilities. Cost and availability will always be a factor.

It is vital that the person with MND, who will have a clear and active mind throughout the illness, is given the means to retain as much control as possible over their life, to play their part in the family life and to pursue their own interests.

So long as work remains enjoyable and important, then it should be continued. Difficulties in travelling, weakness, fatigue, stumbling, loss of manual skills, speech and breathing problems can all be impediments to work. Many of these, however, can be overcome through flexible working hours, travelling by private car, having a parking space that is conveniently close, walking only short distances, avoiding stairs, often simple, obvious ideas, but ones which can make a tremendous impact on a person's ability to continue to work.

The person with MND may need to change from manual to sedentary work with employers taking advantage of their experience for supervision, training and consultancy. They may need a chair with armrests for stability and to make getting up and sitting down easier. There are organisations which can give advice and assistance in this area and they should be contacted at an early stage to make full use of the facilities on offer.

When the decision to finish work is taken then the person with MND will need information on a wide number of issues, many of which they may have no previous knowledge of. The benefits system will perhaps be one of the most pressing at this point; ensuring that they and their family have an adequate income is critical. The role of informant may be taken on by a social worker or doctor, whoever is irrelevant as long as the person with MND and their carer is receiving the appropriate benefits due.[3]

It is clear with MND that the lifespan of the individual can be severely compromised. Every day therefore becomes important and should be rich in experiences for the person and their family. Enid Henke wrote 'I had business and personal friends to attend to and friends who lived a long way away I particularly wanted to see and it was very much a matter of going whilst I could still get in a car and speak clearly enough to make myself understood'.[5] Frustration, anger and anxiety can all be the enemy during hours of inactivity. With the support of everyone and with the advances of technology, old enthusiasms in work, home, recreation and life can be sustained, with concessions being made as strength fades.

The revolution that is taking place in technology is one of the few positive things that we can presently offer to mitigate against the destructive nature of this condition and therefore it should be exploited to the full for the benefit of people with disabilities.

Death and dying

Although everyone is mortal, it is often very difficult to discuss the issues and feelings which can occur at and around death. For most people the idea of death is frightening; there is often a fear of the process of dying or of the unknown.

There are certain needs that must be addressed as the physical deterioration takes place, preferably whilst the person is still able to communicate their more intimate and complex wishes. The first of these is to prepare a will. All too often human mortality is ignored and people refuse to make a will. However, it is important to ensure that plans are clearly defined, to ensure that the person continues to express their choices.

Within the family there is often a need to share what is happening as death draws nearer. The person who is dying needs to feel able to talk about concerns and fears, many of which will be shared by their family. Time is needed to talk issues through and if possible time should be made early in the disease to start this process before time becomes precious.

This preparation can be positive, as the person and family look at their lives together, planning to achieve things that are important to them and tying up loose ends. Family and friends can be seen again, important things can be said and plans can be made. These preparations may not only be for death but for living, visiting or fulfilling a long-standing aim, and growing as a family.

The person with MND may have many fears about the process of death. It is important to allow the person to express their concerns and to answer them as openly as possible. These fears may include:

- Mental incapacitation – dementia is very rare as part of the disease process, although of course a pre-existing dementia is possible.
- Incontinence – the occurrence of incontinence in MND has only been recorded in the later stages of the disease in people on ventilatory support.
- Breathlessness – this in itself is anxiety provoking. Many people with MND experience breathlessness as respiratory muscles weaken. The fear of dying fighting for breath or suffocating is a fear for many. The reality is that the mode of death for a person with a low respiratory reserve is respiratory failure, but this is usually a sudden deterioration over a short period, with little distress, as the intercostal muscles fail and anoxia quickly follows. Severe breathlessness can be controlled pharmacologically.
- A great many people fear choking as the mode of death in MND. However, with careful control of dyspnoea and dysphagia by using medication, choking can usually be reduced and in a large survey of 100 people with MND only one died in a choking attack. However, the person with MND may remain fearful and the issue of choking may need to be discussed openly with them and their carers.
- Pain – many people expect or fear death as a painful event. Pain does occur in about 40 per cent of people with MND, from musculoskeletal causes, muscle spasm or skin pressure due to immobility. These pains can be controlled by the appropriate treatment, for example non-steroidal anti-inflammatory drugs, muscle relaxants or regular analgesia. Passive exercise, careful positioning and appropriate pressure care can ease joints and muscles and improve comfort. Opioid analgesia may be necessary, especially for pressure pain.[6]

The majority of people still believe in a concept of 'God' or an 'ultimate being'. Whilst this can be comforting for some, it may also provoke fears which will need to be expressed and shared with a member of the team caring for the person or with a minister of religion, appropriate to the background and experience of the person.

As can be seen, it is necessary to prepare for the future eventuality during the period of deterioration and while everyone can be involved. This preparation includes both the emotional and social aspects and the prevention of problems by good symptom control.

The decision about where to die will depend upon the individual person and family. Many people wish to stay at home within the family surroundings and this often allows death to be a peaceful experience. Hospice care may be a possibility and here the aim is to provide care, symptom control and support for both the person with MND and their family. If chosen then early introduction to a local hospice and its services, such as home care and day care, may be helpful.

In many cases, death is foreseen and the commonest clinical picture is one of rapid deterioration over a few days, often following an upper respiratory tract infection. There may be a need to recognise this final deterioration and change plans as appropriate.

The care of a person with MND will always need careful planning and close cooperation and communication between the person and their carers. This care needs to be flexible and continue until death so that all can retain a feeling of security and a lessening of fear throughout.[6]

Conclusion

Motor neurone disease is a degenerative condition which acts with such speed it leaves little or no time for emotional adjustment or planning. As yet there is no cure although major research studies are underway and advances in pulmonary care can extend life expectancy considerably. In effect MND severely disables people; it does not kill them.

Intellect is unimpaired, with a few rare exceptions, and diagnosis to death can range from 20 months to 20 years. Personal ambitions remain unaffected and should form the focus of any care package. The average duration of MND without artificial ventilation is 3–5 years. A recent study in the USA places the average at 10 years using artificial ventilation.[7]

Such a diagnosis provides perhaps the greatest emotional challenge both to the individual and to the professionals working in the health and social services that support them. Critical features of services are that they must be client centred, offer continuity and be comprehensive and timely. Key workers should coordinate support services and the emphasis should be on the quality of life. The majority of people prefer to stay in their own homes in the later stages of life when they are very disabled and to die at home.

Advances in technology and an understanding of the disease process mean that there is much that can be done to help people cope with this condition and that effective palliative care programmes and access to specialist services have much to offer in ameliorating its destructive potential.

References

1. Knowles V. Motor neurone disease. In: *Information pack for social and health care professionals*. Northampton: Motor Neurone Disease Association (PO Box 246, Northampton NN1 2PR, UK).

2. Saunders C, Walsh TD, Smith M. A review of 100 cases of motor neurone disease in a hospice. In: Saunders C, Summers DH, Teller N. eds *Hospice: the living idea.* London: Edward Arnold, 1981: 126–46.
3. Cochrane G. In: *The management of motor neurone disease.* Edinburgh: Churchill Livingstone, 1987.
4. George J, Jones C, Le Patourel J. MND – The role of the speech therapist. In: *Information pack for social and health care professionals.* Northampton: Motor Neurone Disease Association (PO Box 246, Northampton NN1 2PR, UK), 1989.
5. Henke E. Motor Neurone Disease – a patient's view. *BMJ* 1968; 4: 765–6.
6. Oliver D. MND – death and dying. In: *Information pack for social and health care professionals.* Northampton: Motor Neurone Disease Association (PO Box 246, Northampton NN1 2PR, UK), 1990/1.
7. Oppenheimer T. At *5th International Symposium on ALS/MND.* Noordwijk, Holland (personal communication) 1994.

Further reading

Kelly M, Cats M. Hospice care in motor neurone disease. *Nursing Standard* 1994; 9: No 9.
Oliver D. *Motor neurone disease.* Exeter: Royal College of General Practitioners, 1989.
Sedal L. The management of motor neurone disease. *Patient Management* 1987; February.

5

Day care for patients with AIDS or HIV disease

Veronica Moss

Introduction

Historical perspective

The first day care facilities for patients with AIDS or HIV disease were developed at hospitals in America in the mid–1980s, in particular in San Francisco and New York. This was in response to the increasing pressure for beds that was developing as more and more patients were being admitted for acute care, and subsequently requiring follow up treatment with intravenous drugs. As the parameters of this new disease were being identified during the early 1980s, new and sometimes very aggressive intravenous therapies were being developed to deal with the frightening opportunistic infections, such as *Pneumocystis carinii* pneumonia which so frequently proved fatal in the early days. The epidemic form of Kaposi's sarcoma which became dramatically evident, especially among gay men, also required new regimes of chemotherapy and/or radiotherapy.

The fear, prejudice and stigma surrounding the disease also led to isolation and rejection of those infected, not only by the public but also by many health care professionals. This meant that sexually transmitted diseases (STD) clinics in the main centres, such as San Francisco, New York and London, became the focus points for many patients requiring care and treatment, and also for the 'worried well'. It came as a natural progression that centres were developed which could provide a social focus, with counselling and other emotional support, together with access to medical care, intravenous therapies and blood transfusions on a day basis for those who were ill. The staff were there by choice and developed an understanding of the issues and problems patients faced, and also increased their expertise in AIDS care. Many patients volunteered to take part in research trials for new treatment regimes and an information network developed amongst patients about possible new therapies. Patients attending these centres became increasingly aware and educated about the disease and developed networks through which information about research and new possibilities were spread. They inevitably also became very aware of the possible problems which lay in store for them as their disease progressed and would clutch at any straw of hope for this devastating and life-threatening condition. In America and the UK the majority of those affected were gay men, many of whom were very articulate, able to demand attention and to set up self-help organisations. The medical and nursing professions were made to rethink much of their practice in relation to patient care, and governments were challenged about discriminatory policies and laws.

As numbers of infected people increased, as treatments improved and the introduction of zidovudine and prophylaxis reduced mortality rates and lengthened median survival times,[1] so it became necessary to develop better support for patients in the community. Day care centres and home support teams began to be developed which would enable treatments to be given at home or on an out-patient basis. Social and counselling support became an integral part of the services offered in the larger urban centres such as London, New York and San Francisco. In some European countries such as France, Spain and Italy, the concept of a day hospital for the investigation and treatment of patients with HIV-related problems was also explored and has been shown to reduce the need for hospitalisation and in-patient care.[2,3] A number of different models are described and will be discussed below.

Models of day care in HIV/AIDS

Hospital-based therapeutic model

This model was first introduced at San Francisco Hospital in California to deal with the increasing numbers of patients requiring intravenous therapies and blood transfusions for whom admission to hospital was not necessary or was too expensive. Other centres in America and Europe found the model effective in reducing the number of in-patient admissions while providing support for people living at home through the social networks that developed.[3,4,5] A well-known example of such a model in London is the Kobler Centre at Chelsea and Westminster Hospital.

Drop-in centres for HIV-positive people

The drop-in centre developed initially as the result of self-help groups such as Body Positive setting up information, advice and social support centres. These tended, in the early days, to be dominated by gay men, but as the epidemic developed the centres ensured that others, especially women, were made to feel welcomed and included. Some, for example, devoted a day or special activities to women. Women also set up their own support centres, such as one run by Positively Women. London Lighthouse purchased an old school building and refurbished it completely to set up a large social support drop-in centre with a restaurant open to the public, and a number of activities, such as counselling and complementary therapies, on offer. They also incorporated a residential unit providing respite and convalescent care for people with AIDS or HIV-related problems. More recently, the Globe Centre has opened in east London as a large drop-in centre.

Palliative day care for symptomatic or ill patients

This is the model developed by Mildmay Mission Hospital in the East End of London in conjuction with its palliative care in-patient units and family care centre. This model provides for a set number of patients to attend daily, having been referred from acute centres, from Mildmay's in-patient units, by general practitioners, social workers or community nurses. Transport is provided to bring patients to the centre and to take them home again at the end of the day. A relaxed atmosphere pervades, but activities are arranged according to the patients' wishes, such as discussion, drama, outings, art, computer or cooking sessions. All the therapies and care provisions of the hospital are available to the clients attending the day care facility and a doctor attends when necessary at the request of patients or staff, or to give a talk or facilitate discussion about a medical or health-related subject. Other visiting professionals include a solicitor, a chaplain, and a counsellor. Massage, provided by a trained volunteer, is very popular, and other volunteers attend and help with various aspects of the day care facility.

Clinical basics

It is important for those involved in supporting people with AIDS or HIV disease to understand some of the basic clinical facts about HIV. A brief introductory description of the likely progression from HIV infection to advanced HIV-related illness or AIDS will therefore follow. There are many textbooks which detail conditions and therapies for specific conditions for those who wish to deepen their knowledge and understanding, and others that deal with the emotional and social issues in greater depth than is possible in one chapter. Some of these are listed at the end.

The phases through which the infection is likely to progress are as follows:

Acute seroconversion illness

Two to six weeks after initial infection many, but not all, will develop a short, influenza-like illness with fever, arthralgia and, in some instances, a maculopapular rash. There may also be a generalised lymphadenopathy which resolves within weeks. The severity of the rash and the fever have been shown to be prognostic markers for more rapid progression of the disease. It is at this stage that individuals become antibody positive, in other words, they start producing antibodies to HIV. These antibodies are detected by a variety of possible tests, the most common being the ELISA test (enzyme linked immunosorbent assay) which is quick, simple to perform and relatively cheap. However, it must always be confirmed by a more specific test such as the more complex and expensive Western Blot. Once the seroconversion illness is over the individual will return to normal health and will have no distinguishing features to mark him or her out as being HIV antibody positive.

Antibody positive: asymptomatic

Individuals may remain asymptomatic for a variable number of years. Some show no signs of progression even after 10–15 years of follow up; these individuals are being investigated to find out what enables them to deal successfully with the virus. However, the numbers are small and the majority will begin to show signs of progression (e.g. falling CD4 count) 2–6 years after the initial infection. All HIV-positive individuals are infected and carry the virus; they are therefore infectious to others through the normal routes of transmission (*see* 'Sources of infection').

Antibody positive: symptomatic

CD4 molecules on certain cells, such as macrophages and the T-helper lympho-cytes, provide the receptor sites for the virus to gain entrance to the cell. Using the enzyme reverse transcriptase, the viral RNA is incorporated as DNA into the host cell's genetic material. Viral protein is reassembled at a later stage, and new virions extruded through the cell membrane, eventually destroying the cell. Other infected cells self-destruct by a process of apoptosis. The CD4 count is normally above 1200 per cubic millimetre, but as the infection progresses with the con-comitant immunosuppression, it declines while the antigen level rises. The time taken for this process varies considerably; some individuals will progress rapidly to symptomatic disease while others will survive for many years. A recent study in haemophiliac men suggests that up to a quarter of patients will survive for 20 years from seroconversion without developing AIDS.[6] Those who progress to symptomatic disease present in a number of ways, but the usual course is that the individual begins to show signs of ill health including non-specific problems such as fatigue, anorexia, weight loss, diarrhoea and persistent lymphadenopathy. Bacterial and fungal skin infections, seborrhoeic dermatitis, herpes simplex and zoster infections, oral or vaginal candidiasis may occur from time to time. Some patients continue to deteriorate, developing HIV-related conditions, but never one of the AIDS-defining conditions. Patients may die of a chest infection or some other severe illness of advanced HIV disease, but never develop AIDS. Others will present for the first time with a condition that immediately places them in the AIDS category.

AIDS

AIDS is diagnosed when one or more conditions develop which are considered by the Centre for Disease Control to be AIDS defining. As more becomes known about HIV/AIDS the list is up-dated and will differ in certain details in America, Europe and in other parts of the world. HIV disease manifests differently in Africa, for example, than in North America. AIDS indicator diseases include certain opportunistic infections, AIDS-related cancers and HIV encephalopathy or dementia. In North America, a CD4 count below 200 cells per cubic millimetre counts as an indicator for AIDS (see end of chapter for current classification).

Similarities to, and differences from, other life-threatening conditions

All who are faced with a life-threatening condition will have concerns, anxieties and physical problems which, especially towards the end of life, pose similar challenges. The basic principles of good palliative care will apply in most such conditions. The hospice movement has led the way in developing good symptom control principles, and in recognising the need to provide for emotional, social and spiritual care, as well as physical care for the patient and all who are close to him or her. The same basic approach also applies in the care of someone with advanced HIV or AIDS, but there are a number of significant differences which must be taken into account when planning to provide services for such a patient.

Differences from cancer care

Table 5.1 Common features of AIDS which are likely to differ from those of the terminally ill patient with cancer

1.	Predominantly younger age group (0–5 years; 16–49 years).
2.	Multisystems disease with multiple problems:

    • blindness
    • paralysis
    • neuropathy
    • dementia
    • myopathy
    • skin disorders
    • severe diarrhoea
    • chest infections

3. Misery of many coexisting diagnoses.
4. Polypharmacy.
5. Sudden, dramatic changes in condition – difficulty in identification of terminal phase.
6. Need for very active palliation or maintenance, e.g. with IV infusions and treatment of opportunistic infections.
7. Lengthy dying process – at times patients may be unconscious for a week or more.
8. Changing pattern of disease and treatment.
9. Patient awareness relating to the disease and its treatment.
10. Isolation, stigma and lack of compassion for patient and family.
11. Lack of family and support structures.
12. Housing problems including homelessness, inappropriate accommodation and need for supervision.

From: *Palliative care for people with AIDS*, Sims and Moss, 1995.

Sources of infection

HIV is usually transmitted in the following ways:

• Through sexual intercourse, anal or vaginal, where infected semen or vaginal fluid is present.
• As a result of infected blood gaining entrance:
  – via a blood transfusion or through blood products e.g. factor VIII
  – through a breach in the skin or mucosa
  – through the conjunctiva
  – via a hollow needle e.g. drug users sharing 'works'.
• From mother to child:
  – *in utero*
  – during birth
  – through breast milk.

The transplantation of infected organs may also lead to transmission.

Issues and preoccupations

People with AIDS or HIV-related health problems are preoccupied by a number of issues, some of which may be similar to those facing any incurable or terminal illness, some of which are specific to this client group. The clients do not form a cohesive group, of course, they come from every walk of life and occupation. However, there are a number of subgroups which have their own particular problems while all patients with HIV or AIDS have certain anxieties or issues in common. Each individual or family deals with these issues in their own unique way, and it is essential not to categorise people or to make assumptions about behaviour. Anyone planning to set up services for people with HIV or AIDS would do well first to spend time seeking to understand the social, emotional and spiritual issues, as well as the physical health problems with which they are likely to be faced. Cultural attitudes and boundaries are important to understand and to respect as well.

Confidentiality

The fear, ignorance and stigma that still surround this virus and those affected by it makes this one of the most important issues with which to come to grips when planning services or dealing with individuals who are infected. Patients or clients will often be fearful of attending a centre which identifies them as having AIDS. They may also be afraid of giving permission for medical information to be shared even with other doctors, for example a general practitioner, or with other health-care professionals. Many have experienced the results of 'leaked' information – antagonism, fear, rejection, loss of jobs or housing. This means that they are often suspicious and angry because of the treatment they have had at the hands of so-called carers, and that they will be very careful to see only those professionals about whom they have heard, or of whom they have had first-hand experience that they can be trusted.

Anxieties about health problems

Those patients or clients who have seen friends or family members become ill and die as a result of HIV or AIDS will naturally be anxious about their own health. Minor symptoms may become cause for great concern and some become so depressed at the possible future problems that they may become suicidal. Multiple bereavements in a short space of time may give little time for grieving and some will develop clinical depression or other psychiatric problems as a result.

Anxieties about health will include, for most, worries about prognosis, the meaning of certain symptoms or diagnoses, the latest CD4 count, and the side-effects of drugs, especially those that are being discussed in the latest newspaper reports about HIV-related treatments. Many become very knowledgeable about the latest research, and have contacts in other countries which keep them informed about new anti-viral drugs, herbal treatments and ideas about how to boost the immune system. They often know more than the health care professionals, especially those who are not usually involved in HIV/AIDS care, and are likely to challenge advice or proffered treatment.

Acceptance

Most HIV-infected individuals have experienced rejection, stigmatisation and isolation as a result of their infection, if it is known, or because of their lifestyle, for example, that of a drug user or a gay man. Those who have been infected as a result of treatment for haemophilia may have disabilities as a result of bleeds into joints over many years and have had years of hospital experience, especially on an out-patient basis. Acceptance of the person by carers can transform lives that have become lonely and despairing, or full of anger and suspicion.

Financial and housing problems

The majority of patients will have financial worries. Patients whose illness is advanced will often be debilitated and weak, or they may have some disability or be developing signs of dementia, making it impossible to continue working. They will be living on their savings or on welfare benefits, if available, or will need family or friends to provide for them. Refugees or illegal immigrants will be preoccupied with financial worries, anxieties about their status, or about being found out and deported. Some, who may be students or legitimate visitors, may have become ill during the visit and are alone and frightened, with few, if any, family members available to help or support them. Housing may be a major problem.

Group bonding and trust

The issue of trust and confidentiality may be one reason why some clients appear to be 'cliquey', becoming very involved and friendly with each other. However, they may not easily welcome newcomers into the group. It takes time to develop trust amongst a group of people, and many clients will have had experiences that have made them suspicious of health care professionals, especially doctors or ministers of religion, or of individuals who do not come from the same background or lifestyle as their own. Thus, when a group has become established, a newcomer may feel excluded, find it difficult to make friends and give up. There are often strong feelings of being 'bonded' to a particular way of life or viewpoint. Some gay men have very strong political agendas and are articulate and motivated to take part in activist demonstrations; others will not wish to be involved and prefer not to be too closely associated with them. Patients with haemophilia may feel angry and blame gay men for their infection and, if they are also heterosexual, may have difficulties mixing with gay men. Drug users come from all walks of life, but may have problems with living within the boundaries set by the centre or the group. Women from countries where they do not normally mix with men to discuss personal issues may find their needs are not catered for in a mixed group.

Women and children

A woman with one or more children will mostly be preoccupied with their health, their schooling, clothing, feeding and happiness. When she herself is ill, she will be worried about who will care for them. Women often come forward for treatment themselves at a late stage because they have been fulfilling their caring role for other members of the family. In Britain and the USA women will often be very unhappy about their children being taken into care, i.e. into a care home or for fostering. This is often expressed as their greatest fear, other than illness and death. Many women will be single mothers, their partner having abandoned them when the infection became known, or as a result of a mutually agreed separation or divorce. Where heterosexual transmission is the norm, and equal numbers of men and women are infected, the woman may have been widowed as a result of HIV disease, or of any other of the many causes of premature death. In developing countries there is not usually any welfare system to support such women, and the struggle for survival on a day to day basis may be the most important issue. The children will often have to help with work in the fields to grow food or cash crops, and schooling has to be abandoned. The woman may have no alternative way of earning money to feed her family other than through prostitution.

Planning a day care facility

There are a number of considerations to take into account when planning a day care facility for patients or clients with HIV or AIDS. These include, first, a decision about the client groups to be served, at what stage of the disease they are likely to be, the cost implications of the model to be developed and the facilities to be offered. It is essential to research the likely client groups, and to develop an understanding of their interests and their perception of their own needs if the facility is to be successful. A survey was conducted at Mildmay, using an anonymous questionnaire distributed to existing clients and referring professionals, including doctors. The results showed that the perceptions of need of the two groups were often at variance with each other. What the clients wanted was not always what the professionals thought they wanted.[7] Clients varied greatly as to their expectations and their likes and dislikes.

Client group

The type of facility offered will depend on the clients and their particular needs. HIV-positive individuals who have no specific health concerns, but who want an information resource and a social centre, will require less medical and nursing input than clients who have symptomatic disease or AIDS. Most women will be looking for facilities where their children can be left in safety. Clients who are disabled or very debilitated will require the facility to have wheelchair access, handrails in corridors and toilets with appropriate facilities. These points may be self evident when dealing with obviously ill or disabled people, but it should be remembered that clients become attached to a centre and its staff, but that their disease is likely to progress so that facilities that were suitable for an ambulant and relatively fit person may be unusable by someone who has progressed to the advanced stages of the disease.

Siting and access

Siting and access to the centre will play an important part in determining how successful it is. Some clients will be very unlikely to attend a centre that identifies them as having AIDS if the entrance to it is easily seen from the street. However, if it is hidden inside a large building such as a hospital or a church which is known to have other functions the anxiety will be allayed and use encouraged. Others will not be bothered by that aspect but will only use a centre that is easily accessible by public transport, unless transport is provided.

Staffing

The staffing will depend on the client groups, the stage of the disease and the model chosen. Nurses and doctors would be required if clients are to be given medical treatments, such as:

- IV infusions of gancyclovir or foscarnet (maintenance treatment of cyto-megalovirus retinitis);
- blood transfusions (e.g. for anaemia in patients on zidovudine);
- nebulised pentamidine as prophylaxis against *Pneumocystis carinii* pneumonia (PCP);
- wound dressings (e.g. patients with Kaposi's sarcoma which has ulcerated).

Symptom–control advice and treatment may be a useful service to the client as well as to the referring doctors. However, the relationship with the GP and the acute centre will have to be determined and, perhaps, negotiated. Many clients will be particularly interested in complementary therapies, massage for example, and staff or volunteers who are able to offer them will be found to be very popular. Access to specialist advice is essential, and it would be helpful to have made arrangements for clients attending the centre to have the possibility of being admitted for acute or respite care should this be required urgently. Liaison and communication with appropriate hospital or hospice facilities should be maintained to ensure continuity of care.

Because of the complex nature of HIV/AIDS it may be advisable to include at least one nurse in the core staffing. If it is decided not to offer medical or nursing skills, other staff with an interest in this client group will be needed. Social workers, occupational therapists, counselling and pastoral staff may be very successful in meeting the non-medical needs of the clients. Dietetic advice is important and volunteers may be very helpful, adding a dimension of normality (i.e. not health related) to the activities.

The importance of confidentiality must be understood by all staff and volunteers.

Activities and facilities

Once the client group has been established, it is important to research their needs and wishes in relation to a day care facility. Do they want a social drop-in centre with no structured activities? Would they like access to legal advice, counselling, or medical care? Do they prefer a structured programme? If so, in what activities or topics would they be interested? Do certain members of the group wish to have information or advice about 'safer sex' in relation to partners who may not be infected? Are there issues around sexuality that need to be discussed? Would they like to have regular medical check-ups and symptom–control advice? How would these relate to their on-going follow-up at their acute out-patient clinic? Where does the GP fit in? Would they respond to the provision of facilities that would enable them to develop new or maintain existing skills, such as computers, needlework, art materials? Would certain subgroups (for example, women) within the whole clientele like to have time to themselves? If so, what would be their particular concerns? Would it be helpful to provide a nursery? Against the answers to these questions has to be considered the likely cost of staffing the centre and providing the necessary facilities.

Transport

The question of transport may be very important when the clients are in the more advanced stages of HIV-related illness or debility. The catchment area will then also have to be determined, and it is necessary to recognise that patients with AIDS or HIV disease may not always be able to keep routine appointments because of the unpredictable nature of the illness. Sudden and dramatic changes may occur, or the patient simply feels very fatigued on waking up. The driver may then arrive and find the client has been admitted to hospital or is too tired to get up. Patients with HIV encephalopathy (or AIDS dementia) may become confused or behave bizzarely or abusively. Staff, in particular drivers, will require training in how to handle such situations. Lifting and handling techniques are another important aspect of training for anyone who is involved in picking people up from their homes and taking them back. Many will be anxious about infection through vomiting, diarrhoea and bleeding, should any occur during the journey and will require instructions as to how to deal with such occurrences.

Staff training

The level of training that will be required by staff and volunteers will depend on their role, their existing knowledge and the type of care that is being offered. All personnel will require some understanding of the disease itself, of infection control and confidentiality issues, and most will need to explore their attitudes and think constructively about the words they use and their body language when meeting someone for the first time. Anyone with HIV is likely to be particularly sensitive to any suggestion or sign of aversion, fear, prejudice or shock. Some may try to shock in order to judge how far they may trust the person concerned. The use of specific words, in a Western setting, may be understood to indicate a certain ignorance about HIV or AIDS, or judgmentalism or homophobia. The words 'victim' or 'sufferer' are sometimes felt to be condescending or derogatory; 'homosexual' instead of 'gay' may be seen as homophobic or indicating lack of sympathy and understanding; 'family' may be taken to exclude a partner of the same sex; drug 'addict' instead of 'user' is thought to indicate judgmentalism. For those who have never been rejected and marginalised by society, this may seem an unjustified sensitivity, but it is easy to accept when the reality of the stigma and prejudice that most individuals with HIV or AIDS have experienced is understood.

It is also important to consider the 'doctor–patient' and 'nurse–patient' relationship in training. Many individuals with HIV are creative and professional people who are used to being in control, and expect to make the decisions about their treatment or other activities. Many are very articulate and well-read and will know as much, if not more, than the doctor or nurse about HIV and AIDS. They are likely to challenge any suggestions of treatment or investigation with which they are not in agreement or which they do not understand.

Infection control

In any health care setting providing for clients and patients with HIV or AIDS, clear policies and guidelines must be developed relating to the handling of potentially infectious material, such as blood. Health care professionals who are involved in invasive procedures should follow guidelines issued by the Department of Health[8] for protection from infection by hepatitis viruses and HIV. In summary, these are:

- Always use gloves whenever dealing with blood or body fluids;
- Cover any cuts or abrasions of the skin with waterproof plasters;
- Never resheath a needle using both hands;
- Always place used needles and syringes into a 'sharps' container immediately; if there is any chance of recycling, then the container should have a 1:10 solution of bleach to cover any disposed needles or syringes; container should not be filled above two-thirds to avoid injury to personnel disposing of 'sharps' and should be incinerated or buried once full;
- Always handle a scalpel safely, pointing the blade away from yourself and others;
- Always dispose of used sharp instruments safely, preferably so that they cannot be recycled; if they may be, then always sterilise infected material with 1:10 solution of bleach (sodium hypochlorite) or 70 per cent alcohol, or by boiling or autoclaving;
- If splashing is likely during any procedure, then goggles or spectacles should be worn.

The virus is easily destroyed at temperatures above 56°C as well as by bleach or alcohol as above.

NEVER LEAVE NEEDLES OR SYRINGES WHERE CHILDREN MAY REACH THEM.

Infection control in any other situation is a simpler matter, as there is no evidence from anywhere in the world that transmission is possible in any social setting. Transmission from cutlery, china, toilet seats, through the air or by normal touch is not a problem, nor is hugging or kissing as a means of greeting or in giving comfort. All staff should know where gloves (normal household or surgical varieties) are kept and should use them for mopping up any spillages involving body fluids. Bleach, in the form of a 1:10 solution of sodium hypochlorite, should be available to soak materials used for mopping up purposes and it is helpful to have bleach in the form of granules (such as 'Precept') available to cover a spillage for 20 minutes prior to cleaning up from the floor or other surface.

Other infections

Patients with oozing sores or herpes simplex skin infections should be encouraged to avoid touching the infected area. Other patients may be at risk of contracting the infection if the organisms are transferred on someone's hands. Good standards of hand hygiene should be maintained at all times by both staff and patients. Patients with 'open' pulmonary tuberculosis should avoid being in close proximity to other immuno-compromised patients until they have received treatment for an appropriate period to prevent nosocomial spread and all staff should be Mantoux tested, and if necessary given a BCG vaccination. The specialist in charge of the treatment should be consulted as to the 'safety' of mixing with other patients.

Infection-control policies for a nursery or creche where some of the children may be HIV positive should be developed with a paediatrician to ensure that they are protected as far as possible from infections such as measles, chicken-pox and other childhood illnesses.

Mixing HIV with other conditions

A number of traditional cancer hospices are now admitting patients with AIDS or HIV-related conditions very successfully. However, a number of issues will have to be considered when planning to incorporate services for cancer or other non-AIDS patients with AIDS and HIV. Some of these issues have already been mentioned above, and will be dealt with briefly.

Attitudes and confidentiality

The attitude of staff has already been dealt with above, but it is also important to consider the attitude of other clients and their families. There may be fear, anger, or rejection when it becomes known that someone has AIDS, and other clients may refuse to attend. The other clients may be afraid of drinking and eating from the same china and with the same cutlery. They may worry about using the same toilet facilities. They may be hostile to the person concerned, but even if they are not, there may be the lurking fears and anxieties that make it difficult to mix easily. Education and example from staff will deal with these worries, but that takes time. The staff will undoubtedly keep confidentiality, but can this be demanded, or expected, of other clients? What if the information is 'leaked' to the press? There is still a prurient interest in this disease and much distress may be caused to the patient and his/her partner and family.

Staff knowledge of HIV/AIDS

It is difficult to maintain adequate knowledge of the latest research and developments in treatment protocols when staff are dealing with only a small number of patients with AIDS or HIV-related conditions. It is important to ensure that staff are kept up to date as the field of HIV/AIDS is still rapidly developing, and patients will often keep in touch with what is going on, and wish to ask advice.

HIV encephalopathy or AIDS dementia complex

Approximately 30 per cent of patients with advanced HIV disease will develop signs of AIDS dementia. The early signs include short-term memory loss, intermittent confusion and personality changes. Some patients will become disinhibited, displaying bizarre or unusual behaviour, not realising that it is unacceptable or disturbing to others. The intermittent confusion may result in severe anxiety when the patient is lucid, realising that he has been confused and may become so again. The loss of short-term memory and confusion means that the individual requires 24-hour supervision for his or her own safety as well as that of others. As the disease progresses ataxia, tremors, limb weakness and other diffuse neurological signs will develop, finally resulting, in the end stages, in severe or total dementia, urinary and faecal incontinence, grand mal attacks and a complete dependence on carers. It may be possible to accommodate patients with the early signs of dementia in a day care setting, but they may require more supervision than the other clients, who may be frightened or resentful. Other clients who are HIV positive or have AIDS may become unhappy and anxious as they watch the progress, relating it to their own possible future. Those who have other conditions than AIDS may find the unpredictable behaviour difficult to handle, and may become angry or irritated by the constant repetition that is necessary when talking to the person with dementia. Communication may be impossible in the more advanced stages of the disease and the condition of the person will be distressing to all. Much thought and planning would have to go into mixing such patients with others, whether HIV positive or not. It would also be important to give thought to what ratios of clients/patients with certain conditions it would be appropriate to include, as it would have a bearing on the staffing required. One or two in a group of ten may be manageable but more than that would be very difficult.

Psychiatric problems

These are common amongst patients with HIV or AIDS, although research would indicate that psychiatric problems may not always be directly related to the infection.[9] The commonest problems are psychosocial, with adjustment disorders, anxiety and depression relating to the diagnosis and the problems arising therefrom. Many patients will have pre-existing neuroses or personality problems. Suicidal behaviour does not appear to be more common than in patients with other life-threatening conditions, although euthanasia is frequently an issue. Those at greatest risk are individuals lacking in social support, injecting drug users and partners and relatives of those infected, especially small children

Psychotic disorders including hypomania and schizophrenia-like illnesses have an uncertain aetiology,[10] but sometimes appear to be associated with developing dementia or an acute episode of illness. It is important to ensure that psychiatric advice is available and that staff on the day care centre are trained to cope with patients displaying unusual behaviour. Policies should also be developed which give staff guidelines about dealing with aggression as, although the majority of patients will not be violent, an occasional person will become verbally or physically aggressive.

Conclusion

Mixing patients with different diagnoses in a day care centre will demonstrate that there is no risk of transmitting HIV in a social setting and some patients with HIV-related problems will much prefer to be in such a day care facility, away from constant reminders of HIV and feeling part of the 'normal' world as they might express it. Other clients may have difficulties in mixing with an HIV-positive person, but once the prejudice and fear that exists around HIV is lifted, many have found friendship and support in such situations.

However, many people with HIV or AIDS wish to meet with others who are 'in the same boat', and feel safer if attending a centre that is known to be staffed by professionals who are trained and knowledgeable about the disease. Many have common issues and concerns which they need to discuss or they wish to find others who are dealing with the same problems. In many large Western cities networks of support have developed from such centres which have provided a creative forum for achieving further care or for political activity which has influenced decisions at government level. In countries such as Uganda where resources are very limited, day care is providing one effective way of supporting patients with AIDS. For example, The AIDS Support Organisation (TASO) has set up counselling and day care centres which have influenced the development of care throughout Africa and in other developing countries. It is possible to develop cost-effective and supportive palliative day care as one important element of the response that is needed to the greatest challenge to health care in this century.

Acknowledgements

The author thanks the following people for their help in discussion about day care in HIV/AIDS:

Alec Kemp, Day Centre Manager, Mildmay Mission Hospital.
Henrietta Gammell, Quality Facilitator, Mildmay Mission Hospital.
Individual patients and clients.
Thanks also to Eileen Haken for typing the manuscript.

References

1. Peters BS, Beck EJ, Coleman DG *et al.* Changing disease patterns in patients with AIDS in a referral centre in the UK; the changing face of AIDS. *BMJ* 1991; **302**: 203–7.
2. Visco CV, Arici C, Mastrilli F, Ippolito G, Guzzanti E. Measuring the output of hospital care services for HIV infected patients in Italy; methodological and empirical improvements *Int Conf AIDS* 1993; **9**(2): 921 (abstract No. PO-D28-4220).
3. Polo RM, Mendez E, Mejias MM, Algors J, Laguna F, Soriano V, Gonzalez-Lahoz J. Experience in a daycare unit for HIV infected patients. *Int Conf AIDS*, 1992; **8**(3): 212 (abstract No. PuD 9079).
4. Illig JM. AIDS day health care – a new model of therapeutic community. *Int Conf AIDS* 1992; **8**(2):D520 (abstract No. POD5787).
5. Cowan J, Kloser PC. The outpatient infusion clinic as a model of care. *Int Conf AIDS* 1992; **8**(2):D476 (Abstract No. POD 5537).
6. Phillips AN, Sabin CA, Elford J, Bofill M, Janossy G, Lee CA. Use of CD4 lymphocyte count to predict long term survival free of AIDS after HIV infection. *BMJ* 1994; **309**: 309–13.
7. Gammell H. A review of day care services at Mildmay Mission Hospital (unpublished).
8. HMSO. *Guidance for clinical health care workers: protection against HIV and hepatitis viruses.* London: HMSO, 1990.
9. Catalan J. *HIV infection and mental health care.* Geneva: WHO Second Report, 1993.
10. Catalan J. Psychotic illnesses in HIV disease. *Abstracts of the Neurosciences of HIV International Meeting*, Amsterdam, 1992.

Further reading

Advisory Council on the Misuse of Drugs. *AIDS and drug misuse*. London: HMSO, 1988.

Claxton R, Harrison A. *Caring for children with HIV and AIDS*. London: Edward Arnold, 1990.

HMSO. Guidance for clinical health care workers: protection against HIV and hepatitis viruses. London: HMSO, 1990.

Kirkpatrick B. *AIDS: sharing the pain*. London: Darton, Longman and Todd, 1988.

Marcetti A, Lunn S. *A place of growth*. London: Darton, Longman and Todd, 1993.

Miller D. *Living with AIDS and HIV*. Basingstoke: Macmillan, 1987.

Pratt R. *AIDS: a strategy for nursing care*, 3rd edn. London: Edward Arnold, 1991.

Robertson AR. *Heroin, AIDS and society*. Sevenoaks: Hodder & Stoughton, 1987.

Royal College of Nursing. *Nursing guidelines on the management of patients in hospital and the community suffering from AIDS*. London: Sentari Press, 1986.

Sims R, Moss VA. *Palliative care for people with AIDS*, 2nd edn. London: Edward Arnold, 1995.

Appendix

Table 5.2 Classification of HIV disease

AIDS indicator disease	Definitive or presumptive	Definitive diagnostic method(s) or presumptive diagnostic criteria
Bacterial infections, recurrent, in a child aged less than 13 years	Definitive	Culture, antigen detection, multiple or CSF microscopy.
Candidiasis, trachea, bronchi or lungs	Definitive	Gross inspection at endoscopy/ post-mortem or by microscopy (histology or cytology).
Candidiasis of oesophagus	Definitive	Gross inspection at endoscopy/ post-mortem or by microscopy (histology or cytology).
	Presumptive	Recent onset retrosternal pain on swallowing or radiological evidence and confirmed oral or pharyngeal candidiasis.
Cervical carcinoma, invasive	Definitive	Histology.
Coccidioidomycosis, disseminated or extrapulmonary	Definitive	Microscopy, culture of, or antigen detection in, affected tissue.

Table 5.2 (*Continued*)

AIDS indicator disease	Definitive or presumptive	Definitive diagnostic method(s) or presumptive diagnostic criteria
Cryptococcosis, extrapulmonary	Definitive	Microscopy, culture of, or antigen detection in, affected tissue.
Cryptosporidiosis, with diarrhoea for over 1 month	Definitive	Stool microscopy.
Cytomegalovirus retinitis	Presumptive	Loss of vision and characteristic appearance on serial ophthalmoscopy, progressing over several months.
Cytomegalovirus disease (onset after age 1 month) not in liver, spleen or nodes	Definitive	Culture lung tissue, microscopy (histology or cytology), antigen or nucleic acid detection.
Encephalopathy (dementia) due to HIV	Definitive	HIV infection or disabling cognitive and/or motor dysfunction, or milestone loss in a child, with no other causes by CSF examination, brain imaging or post-mortem.
Herpes simplex: ulcers for 1 month or bronchitis, pneumonitis, oesophagitis (onset after age 1 month)	Definitive	Culture, microscopy of, or antigen detection in, affected tissue.
Histoplasmosis, disseminated or extrapulmonary	Definitive	Microscopy, culture of, or antigen detection in, affected tissue.
Isosporiasis, with diarrhoea for over 1 month	Definitive	Microscopy (histology or cytology).
Kaposi's sarcoma	Definitive Presumptive	Microscopy (histology or cytology). Characteristic erythematous/ violaceous plaque-like lesion on skin or mucous membrane.
Lymphoid intersitial pneumonia and/or pulmonary lymphoid hyperplasia in a child aged less than 13 years	Definitive Presumptive	Microscopy (histology or cytology). Diffuse bilateral reticulonodular pulmonary interstitial infiltrates for over 2 months and no pathogen identified and no antibiotic response.
Lymphoma: Burkitt's or immunoblastic or primary in brain*	Definitive	Microscopy (histology or cytology).

Table 5.2 (*Continued*)

AIDS indicator disease	Definitive or presumptive	Definitive diagnostic method(s) or presumptive diagnostic criteria
Mycobacteriosis: (including extrapulmonary TB) disseminated*	Definitive	Culture.
	Presumptive	AFB (species not identified by culture) on microscopy of stool specimen or normally sterile body fluid/tissue, not lungs, skin, cervical or hilar nodes.
Mycobacteriosis: pulmonary tuberculosis*	Definitive	Culture or other definitive demonstration of *M. tuberculosis* infection.
	Presumptive	Clinical diagnosis, with or without AFB on microscopy, resulting in initiation of anti-TB therapy.
Pneumocystis carinii pneumonia	Definitive	Microscopy (histology or cytology).
	Presumptive	Recent onset dyspnoea on exertion or dry cough, and diffuse bilateral interstitial infiltrates on CXR and pO_2 <70 mmHg (9.3 kPa) and no evidence of bacterial pneumonia.
Pneumonia recurrent within a 12-month period	Definitive	Microscopy (histology or cytology).
	Presumptive	CXR or clinical diagnoses of two distinct episodes of pneumonia.
Progressive multifocal leukoencephalopathy	Definitive	Electron microscopy, antigen detection in brain or urine, antibody in serum or CSF.
Salmonella (non-typhoid) septicaemia, recurrent	Definitive	Culture.
Toxoplasmosis of brain onset after age 1 month	Definitive	Microscopy (histology or cytology), mouse inoculation, tissue culture.
	Presumptive	Recent onset focal neurological abnormality or reduced level of consciousness, and mass effect lesion on scan, and serological evidence or specific therapy response.
Wasting syndrome due to HIV	Definitive	Weight loss (over 10% baseline) with no no other cause, and 30 days or more of either diarrhoea or weakness with fever.

*Full case definition and notes on AIDS indicator diseases for neoplasms, mycobacteriosis and indicator diseases in children are available from Centre for Disease Statistics and Control (CDSC).
CSF: Cerebrospinal fluid; AFB: Acid fast bacilli; CXR: Chest X-ray.

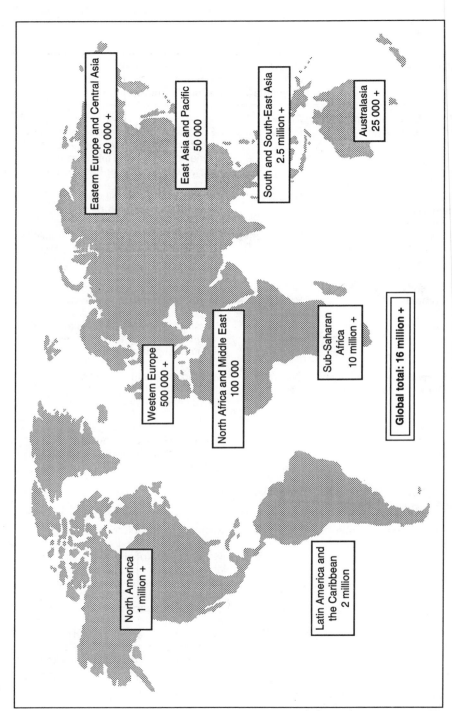

Fig. 5.1 Estimated global distribution of the total adult HIV infections from late 1970s/early 1980s until mid-1994 (WHO).

Eastern Europe and Central Asia
50 000 +

East Asia and Pacific
50 000

South and South-East Asia
2.5 million +

Australasia
25 000 +

Western Europe
500 000 +

North Africa and Middle East
100 000

Sub-Saharan
Africa
10 million +

Global total: 16 million +

North America
1 million +

Latin America and
the Caribbean
2 million

Table 5.3 1993 classification system

Category A:	Acute (primary) HIV infection or asymptomatic HIV infection or persistent generalised lymphadenopathy.
Category B:	Symptomatic with conditions other than those included in categories A or C attributed to HIV infection or which are indicative of a defect in cell-mediated immunity.

For example:
- Bacillary angiomatosis
- Candidiasis, oropharyngeal (thrush)
- Candidiasis, vulvovaginal; persistent, frequent, or poorly responsive to therapy
- Cervical dysplasia (moderate or severe)/cervical carcinoma *in situ*
- Constitutional symptoms, such as fever (38.5°C) or diarrhoea lasting > 1 month
- Hairy leukoplakia, oral
- Herpes zoster (shingles), involving at least two distinct episodes or more than one dermatome
- Idiopathic thrombocytopenic purpura
- Listeriosis
- Pelvic inflammatory disease
- Peripheral neuropathy.

Category C:	Clinical conditions listed in the AIDS surveillance case definition presumptively or definitively diagnosed (see above).

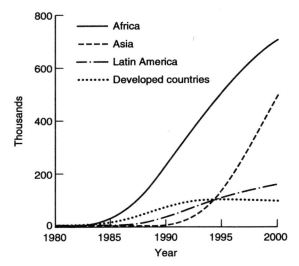

Fig. 5.2 Estimated and projected annual adult AIDS incidences by 'macro' region: 1980–2000 (WHO, 1994).

Part II: Planning

6

Planning and development

Derek Spooner

Where do we start?

One of the most difficult questions to answer is 'What do you mean by day care?' We now have many well-developed services and facilities to meet the needs of the elderly and the mentally ill, and limited developments in other specialities. The idea of providing day care for patients with cancer has been a relatively recent development and was emphasised when a report of a Working Group on Terminal Care was issued by the Department of Health in 1980. Prior to that publication, most developments caring for cancer patients and their families were directed at in-patient care, but with the growing development of domiciliary services and the increasing costs, the direction to expand the service to meet the increasing demands was directed to day care.

Around this time a limited number of day care units had been built or existing buildings had been adapted, but the full range of opportunities which now exist in day care had not been realised, and the facilities were relatively limited. Having been concerned primarily with the building of in-patient units in both the National Health Service and the independent hospice programmes, the introduction of day care into the future plans required a considerable rethink. It was inevitable that not only free-standing day units would be required, but also day units associated with existing facilities.

In order to respond to this need it was necessary to rethink the whole of the planning solution in order to develop facilities which could be incorporated into an acceptable planning philosophy. This philosophy was reflected in the development of Macmillan Green, which will be referred to again later.

To return to the basic question which needs to be asked of anyone contemplating providing day care, the following range of opportunities should be considered. Day care can or should offer:

1. A point of contact between those professionals concerned with the care of cancer patients and others having chronic diseases.
2. Regular medical attention for the review of symptom control, adjustment of medication and other necessary treatments.
3. Provision of the opportunity to discharge in-patients earlier.
4. Nursing care, including general hygiene, specific nursing procedures and counselling.
5. Active physiotherapy.
6. Occupational therapy and assessment.

7. Aids to daily living including assistance in any necessary adaptation to 'home living'.
8. Diversional therapy in the form of handicrafts, group activities, and entertainment.
9. Hairdressing, chiropody and beauty care.
10. A forum to relieve social isolation.
11. A centre to provide support to families and carers.
12. Complementary medicine.
13. Spiritual and emotional support.
14. A resource centre for educational and training purposes (*see* Chapter 11).

This type of day care – all embracing – will make it possible to maintain at home, patients who would otherwise need intermittent or permanent admission to a hospital or hospice or similar. The burden on relatives would be much lighter and admissions precipitated by their exhaustion, avoided.

Thus the prime operational areas comprise:

• Medical care
• Nursing care
• Social care
• Spiritual care
• Management.

Starting the planning process

Planning means two things. Firstly identifying the service need and relating this to the population to be served, modified as appropriate according to the incidence of disease and the apparent trends. At this stage, account should also be taken of any other group of people who have other life-threatening diseases who would benefit from the service to be provided. Over the past 10 or so years a norm of provision of one place per 10 000 population has been applied and has found to be generally satisfactory. The 'place' is defined as: 'one patient, in making one attendance, will occupy one place from say 10.00 a.m. to 4.00 p.m., on one day (Monday to Friday)'. This means that a fifteen-place day unit could care for 75 patients in any one week assuming that each patient makes only one attendance a week. This is obviously a maximum figure and is likely to be somewhat less as there is every indication that each patient attending a day unit tends to make 2.5 attendances a week.

The size of the day unit should not be larger than one able to provide a maximum of twenty places. There are a number of reasons for this, but one of the most critical relates to travelling distances for patients and their families. A twenty-place day unit in theory should serve a population of 200 000 and whether this is in a urban or rural environment, it puts a maximum strain on travel distances. Equally, a larger day unit tends to lose the personal ambience and reduces the level of personal contact between the patients and the staff and volunteers. In practice the most common size of day unit is for around fifteen places.

For service planning, it is recommended that the following factors be established before a final decision is made on the size and location of the day unit:

1. *Demographic*
Population to be served:

(a) Resident population (i.e. those people permanently resident in the area).

(b) Population projection (i.e. the estimated number of people likely to be permanently resident in the area in say 5 or 10 years hence).

(c) Catchment population (i.e. those people living within the area who look to the day centre or who are referred, for care.

2. *Socioeconomic*

(a) Social factors (e.g. deprivation, isolation, and unemployment).

(b) Ethnic considerations (i.e. responding to the particular needs of mixed ethnic communities and taking account of different cultures).

(c) Transport (i.e. awareness of transport problems and possibilities).

3. *Service need*

(a) Extent of proposed service (e.g. cancer patients only).

(b) Standard mortality rates (SMRs).

4. *Resource need*

(a) Day place norms. ⎫ By applying norms* to the population to be
(b) Out-patient norms. ⎬ served estimates of resource need are
(c) Manpower norms. ⎭ derived.

*Norms should be used for guidance only

5. *Current service provision*

(a) Within NHS.

(b) Outside NHS.

(c) Community services.

It is important to assess the level of existing or planned services within the area at an early stage.

The second stage of the planning process is the development of the building scheme whether this be a scheme of adaptation or new build. It is essential that a carefully prepared and complete 'brief' be prepared in order that the design team is fully aware of the intent of the client.

Appendix 1 is a sample questionnaire which endeavours to identify the requirements and aspirations for the future day unit. It is essential that this stage of the planning process is given adequate time and is thoroughly thought through. The information contained will provide not only the design team with the basis of preparing a schedule of accommodation, but also provide the framework for the preparation of operational policies and be the basic data upon which the revenue consequences can be assessed, which of course includes proposed staffing levels.

This basic briefing should be available before consideration is given to the purchase of any existing property. An attractive property set within delightful grounds may not always be the best solution, for so often problems of changing levels, fire protection requirements, doorway widths and the like can result in a very expensive solution. If, however, a property is identified which appears to be suitable, it is wise to undertake an in-depth feasibility study which includes such matters as building surveys, change of use, and initial responses from the local authority's planning department regarding restrictions, covenants, access, etc. Many successful day units have been created in existing properties, but the limitations imposed are sometimes severe and the opportunity for further development and extension of the building is often thwarted by planning restrictions.

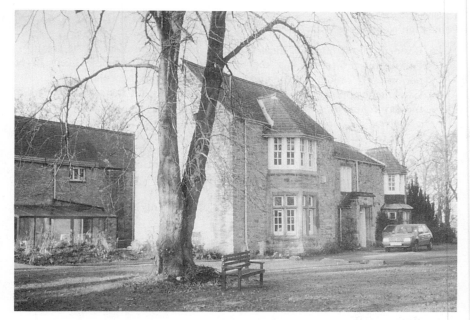

Fig. 6.1 The day unit for St Cuthbert's Hospice, Durham was developed in existing property – a good example of a successful conversion.

The development of a day unit on a green field site has much to commend it. The planning process must be similar to any development and following the initial briefing a schedule of accommodation prepared for the architect to prepare an outline scheme. For such a new building development it is recommended that the first formal report to be prepared by the design team should be a 'project assessment'. This would provide an outline plan for the proposed day unit showing its location, identifying an 'order of costs' and other development matters upon which a strategic decision can be made as to whether or not to proceed with the scheme. If a positive decision is made then to go forward to a full 'feasibility study' which would spell out in detail the total scheme proposals, programme and costs. Following this stage the scheme would then follow the normal design process leading up to tender action and construction.

Where to build

Selection of the site is obviously very important for many reasons. Assuming that planning permission is forthcoming, there is the need to establish the costs associated with developing a given site as these can be very high when the land is situated some distance from the public highway. Apart from access roads and car parking there is the cost of bringing in public utilities i.e. gas, electricity, water and the very important matter of access for patients' relatives and friends and for staff and volunteers. These initial stages of planning are extremely critical and should not be rushed.

The other question which is frequently raised relates to the desirability or otherwise of building the day unit on a hospital site – particularly a district general hospital. There may be advantages in selecting an existing hospital site, but any advantages or disadvantages should be carefully weighed up before making a decision. The location can be so important and the surrounding environment can play a significant part in the rehabilitation of patients. Many factors need to be considered and a full evaluation should be undertaken by way of an option appraisal in order to arrive at the preferred option before proceeding with an in-depth feasibility study.

What should be provided

As it was said earlier, it is important to define the range of activities which are likely to be carried out in the day unit. Based upon experience of planning and developing some thirty day units, many of these being based upon the Macmillan Green planning concept, it is suggested that the following accommodation should be considered:

A central focal point wherein patients can meet, chat and relax

This should be an area where people can undertake a range of activities supported by adequate storage accommodation for equipment and materials. As the focal point of the building, it is essential that this should have a welcoming atmosphere

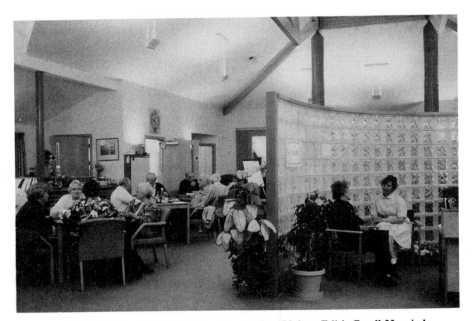

Fig. 6.2 The 'Green' in the Robert Horrell Day Unit at Edith Cavell Hospital, Peterborough. This scheme was completed in July 1987.

and should lead directly from the main reception area. Appendix 2 is a sample activity sheet which sets out the likely range of activities, and it is recommended that for this accommodation and for all rooms throughout the day unit, an attempt should be made at the earliest stage in planning to identify all accommodation required. This should be supported by detailed activity sheets including any specific items of equipment which could have an affect on the area of space required. When planning a new building on a green field site it is obviously easier to determine the functional relationships to this area, but often when an existing building is being considered there is inevitably a need to examine possible opportunities for sharing existing rooms which may need a degree of structural alteration. This is important, as this large activity area is basically the hub of the whole of the day unit and provides that important place for meeting and sharing between patients, families, friends, staff and volunteers.

The chapel

We tend to preach a gospel of total care which includes physical, mental and social, but often the spiritual dimension is forgotten. Bearing in mind that in many parts of the world there are differing requirements for such a spiritual base, in multi-faith societies we need to recognise and respect the very different cultures that exist. It is important at an early stage in planning to reflect the needs of the local community. In many hospices there are chapels which have either been dedicated or consecrated and this often reflects the local Christian tradition and is considered to be a very important facility in the work of the staff. However, in many places it is felt increasingly important to provide non-denominational rooms which can be used by any of the patients and their families for prayer – for a place of peace or just somewhere to sit.

Physiotherapy and occupational therapy

Where a day unit is built on an existing hospital site it is often practical to make arrangements for patients to make use of existing facilities. Such facilities may include aids for daily living such as kitchen, bathroom, bedroom or it may be felt appropriate to include this type of accommodation within the day unit in order to help patients remain active in their own homes by delivering to them a large measure of domestic rehabilitation. Where no hospital facilities exist it is generally recognised that a room is provided for two couch positions in order to include a suitable level of physiotherapy within the day unit itself (*see* Chapter 18). With the benefits of complementary medicine being explored (*see* Chapter 23) it is also possible to offer these within the room identified for physiotherapy. As far as occupational therapy is concerned the range of activities to be offered needs to be carefully defined (*see* Chapters 19 and 20). For many patients the need relates largely to diversional therapy and such other activities which will keep their minds and bodies active rather than seeking a full rehabilitation programme. Again, where facilities are available on a hospital site these should be explored and utilised. One of the main problems which tends to emerge from a fully operational day unit served with active staff and volunteers tends to be the storage of equipment and materials and it is important that adequate provision is made.

Bathrooms and toilet provision

Much has been stated about the great benefits of providing assisted bathroom facilities in day units and I do not think this can be over stressed. Many patients are frail and possibly disabled and are unable to have regular baths in their own homes. Many look forward very much to having the necessary assistance given to them so that they can enjoy and relax in a bath. Many have stated that communication between patient and nurse becomes very relaxed in the privacy of a bathroom and for this reason provision of at least one assisted bathroom in a day unit is essential. There are a number of technical points which require early attention in the planning stage and these should be explored with both the suppliers and the appointed engineers. Equally important is ensuring that adequate space is available for those patients in wheelchairs and this applies equally in the planning and design of toilet facilities. Regarding the number of toilets to be provided, this is often laid down in local regulations and these should be adhered to as a minimum level. In order to retain patients' privacy and dignity, it is always suggested that separate male and female facilities be provided. However, for staff working within the life centre of the day unit, at least one single unisex toilet should be located.

Consultant/treatment

It is important that at an early stage in the planning of facilities that the level of medical input be determined. In some day units the emphasis can be on a general social and support basis, whereas for many others it is important to provide a significant level of medical input by way of out-patient facilities, with particular reference to symptom and pain control. To plan adequately for these services at least one consultant/examination room should be provided, or maybe a consultant room with two adjoining examination rooms. For patients requiring treatments, and this particularly relates to dressings, a separate room should be provided which could double up as a clean utility room in which sterile packs, etc. can be stored. The location for drugs, particularly any scheduled drugs, needs to be agreed with the local pharmacist, police or other authority as appropriate.

Base for primary care team

As the day care unit relates primarily to the community, it is critical that suitable and adequate accommodation is provided as a base for members of the community team. This will include not only domiciliary nurses but also social workers, psychologists and other professionals who will have a role in providing a seamless service from the community through day care leading in many cases to in-patient facilities. Within such accommodation there exists the opportunity for providing a resource centre for all those involved in the caring programme and also for patients and their families. Once again storage is often a problem, as much of the equipment is held in the day room for distribution and subsequent return.

Education

Education is a vital component of the service, and provision should be made for suitable teaching accommodation including at least one seminar room and library. It is important that this be included within the building in order to allow continuing in-service training for staff and volunteer training programmes. Most of these will be multi-professional. Wherever possible such programmes should be integrated with associated hospital and health care programmes and in many cases this will allow the sharing of facilities.

Other accommodation

It will be appreciated that there are many other facilities which need to be provided and these can be classified under three main headings:

1. *Patient orientated*
   - Hairdressing
   - Utility
   - Wheelchair stores
   - Linen and equipment store
   - General store.
2. *Support accommodation*
   - Catering (main kitchen and beverage bars)
   - Non-resident staff changing accommodation
   - Laundry
   - Refuse disposal.
3. *Office accommodation*
   - Medical Director or equivalent
   - Matron or Senior Nurse
   - Administrator (*see* Chapter 8)
   - General office
   - Appeals and fundraising (*see* Chapter 9)
   - Social worker (*see* Chapter 21)
   - Junior medical staff
   - Computer and secretarial staff.

Schedule of accommodation

Table 6.1 in Appendix 3 shows a draft schedule of accommodation which has been the basis of planning of a large number of day units within the UK.

Gardens

Creating the environment within the building is obviously very important, but wherever possible equal attention should be given to the grounds which surround the building (*see* Chapter 7). A mature garden is obviously very desirable, but so often this is not available or the garden may have suffered seriously during the course of construction. There are so many opportunities to benefit both patients and staff when real consideration has been given to the outcome. First, most people can relate to the feeling of peace and space which a well-defined garden can provide. In many cases landscape consultants have been invited to undertake the creation of the garden, but this is not always necessary particularly if an existing garden can be suitably modified to meet the particular needs for the day unit. Areas which can be secluded and developed in order to provide sheltered sitting areas are highly desirable. Equally, many patients appreciate opportunities to make their contribution to the garden, and this means that raised beds and easy access generally should be a prime consideration. A greenhouse and a shed can be very useful points of contact where patients and staff can meet and talk over thoughts and feelings. In one particular scheme, the outcome of providing a greenhouse has been very important. It has provided a place of purpose for patients and has encouraged them to think positively about the future by the simple approach of watching seeds and plants flower and die, and yet in the following year to see those flowers emerge once again.

Vegetable gardening has also proved very useful as patients feel they can make a positive contribution to the hospice by growing their own produce. The possibility of introducing animals into the environment should also be explored. Much has been written about the therapeutic advantages of pets in the hospice; this opportunity should be positively pursued. For many patients and their families and friends, a garden again provides a place where informal counselling and talking can go on away from the immediate proximity of other patients and staff.

Earlier mention was made of the building of a day unit on a green field site. If such a solution is pursued, it is clearly crucial that adequate funding for developing gardens and grounds generally should be included in the preparation of budget costs.

A recommended solution

Shortly after the initial introduction of the day care concept for cancer patients, the author was asked to develop a planning concept which would take account of not only the needs of day care, but also integrating these within the possible whole development for the care of cancer patients, including in-patient facilities, education and support accommodation. This request came from the Cancer Relief Macmillan Fund, London. Working from such an outline brief, the author used the English village green concept although a similar solution in Holland based on the market square was also considered. The first brochure which was published by Cancer Relief in 1987 stated:

> Macmillan Green is a new design and planning concept which meets the particular needs of cancer patients and their carers. Integral to the scheme is 'the Green'. At the centre of the building, the Green is the social and architectural focal point of the building. It is the hub of the patient care community, functioning as a Village Green. It is also a building device giving great flexibility in design.

This has proved to be a very successful design solution and many such units have been built and are now operational in the UK. Equally, the specification of finishes and services has been standardised to a high level without prejudicing cost. Every one of these schemes has been completed within budget.

It is important to state that the various parts of Macmillan Green comprising the Green, day care support, education and in-patient accommodation have been pre-designed, and each of the modules is stored on a computer data base which means that our architects are able to respond quickly to individual projects at a very early stage in the planning process. This means that the lengthy briefing period that often occurs can be reduced, and such savings, in time, lead to substantial cuts in

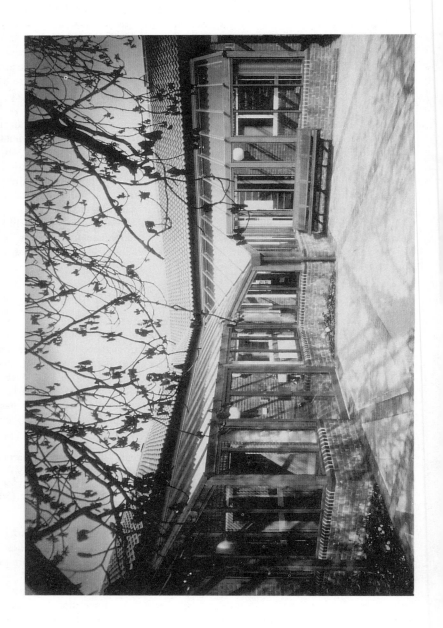

(a)

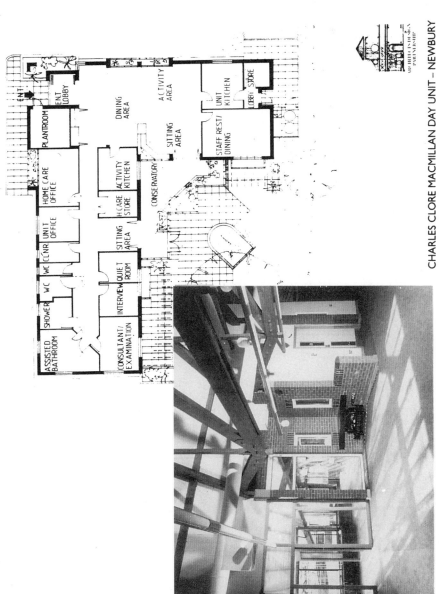

CHARLES CLORE MACMILLAN DAY UNIT – NEWBURY

Fig. 6.3a and b This day unit was one of the first Macmillan Green design buildings which was opened in Newbury in February 1987.

cost. Whilst the various modules have been pre-designed, it is perfectly practical to modify these to meet a particular client's wish if certain variations to a module are requested. Another substantial benefit is the use of pre-set room data sheets. As anybody knows who has been involved in the planning process, the completion of these important documents is very time consuming and frustrating!

Although Macmillan Green was designed particularly for 'new build' it has been found to be very useful in the planning of adaptation and alteration in existing buildings which have been selected for possible day care use. Once again, one must emphasise how very important it is to undertake an initial evaluation of suitability of a building before proceeding with purchase.

The cost

It is obviously difficult to identify actual or comparative costs which can be applied across the globe. In assessing costs for any development, attention should be directed at the total cost. This will include the following:

1. The cost of the building including any tax liability if appropriate.
2. The building on-costs (i.e. the cost of constructing the building on a given site) such as access roads, car parking, fencing, the cost of bringing utility services such as gas, electricity and water to the building from the main highway.
3. The estimated cost for furniture and equipment (a nominal figure for budget purposes of 10 per cent of the estimated building costs has been found generally to give a good guide).
4. Professional fees and expenses for the design team (i.e. architect, quantity surveyor, services engineer and structural engineer) together with others such as interior designer, landscape consultant and any business consultants.
5. To identify an approximate figure to cover legal expenses relating to acquisition of the site/building, service contracts and general legal advice relating to the project.
6. Miscellaneous fees relating to planning control, building regulations or similar.
7. In order to complete a comprehensive budget figure it is recommended that an allowance is also included for commissioning costs. These include for the recruitment of staff, printing of stationery, (including medical records) travelling expenses, removal expenses, etc. It should be remembered that the time allocated for physical commissioning of the building should be short in order to realise the benefit arising from the capital investment. Because of this, most activities relating to the commissioning programme should be planned prior to handover of the building and these activities cost money.

Based on experience with a number of Macmillan Green day units in the UK, quantity surveyors have produced an outline cost statement for day units and this is included as Table 6.3 in Appendix 4.

What else!

Interior design

It has been documented that a well-designed interior care environment can have a positive effect on patients' well-being and that fear of isolation that is often felt can be reduced by pleasing surroundings.

The hospice interior must not be treated as a clinical or 'hospital' environment. Although materials need to conform to health care legislation including cross-infection, fire retardancy and cleaning policies, this need not dictate the design as there are now many materials that can support all this and yet achieve a pleasing relaxed atmosphere.

The use of colour needs to be carefully considered. Soft colours give tranquility to the patients' rooms, but at the same time the day spaces need to be livelier, bright and welcoming, without the use of powerful colours. The lighting scheme should give a flexible solution able to create different moods to suit all activities.

Soft furnishings used in a domestic fashion with fabrics of mixed patterns and textures; soft upholsteries for seating; cushions; drapes and blinds for windows; wall coverings; all help to humanise the spaces.

The coordinated approach must be carried through to the selection of furniture and fittings for the finished interior scheme to be successful.

Operational policies

At the beginning of the planning process it is advisable to spell out clearly how it is expected that the day unit will operate. This document will indicate not only internal organisation but its relationship to the community and other health care facilities available or planned. The main headings to be addressed are:

1. Scope and function
2. Siting and relationship
3. Department layout
4. Space standards for rooms
5. Supporting/linked services
6. Environment and safety
7. Furniture and equipment
8. Management structure
9. Draft staff establishment
10. Outline statement of revenue costs.

Furniture and equipment

Having established the accommodation to be provided, it is recommended that an early start be made on preparing schedules of furniture and equipment. Within the future building contract will be included items which will be supplied and fixed by the contractor. However all 'loose' furniture and equipment needs to be scheduled and costed in order to prepare and complete the total budget cost of the development. A sample schedule for one of the rooms is given in Appendix 5.

Commissioning

To many people the word commissioning implies the moving in of furniture and equipment and staff prior to the operation of the day care unit. However, this is only a small part of 'commissioning' and the process should in fact be commenced at the same time as the building contract is let. Commissioning means bringing the building into use and the planning of this activity should start when the contractor starts, as this will include finalising staffing levels, the recruitment and training of staff and volunteers, preparing procedure guidance, arranging maintenance contracts, publicity, open days for the community and other professionals, the selection of furniture and equipment and many other activities which need to be undertaken in parallel with the building programme. If all these are completed adequately then it should mean that the building can be brought into use well within 1 month of completion. It is therefore desirable that the commissioning programme be identified and initiated at this early stage.

Finally – evaluation

So often we do not benefit from the experience of the past, and in so many cases we tend to redesign the wheel on every occasion. This is not only wasteful in terms of time and resources, but often results in the mistakes of the past being repeated. Many health care projects are evaluated, but rarely are the findings published so that others may benefit. The problem often arises because of the possible scale and complexity of the evaluation. It may be wiser to have a clearly defined, light touch 'design in use' evaluation, as the results can be more clearly understood and are not weighed down with managerial or academic jargon. Very often the most simple observations, once a building has been in use for between 9 and 12 months, can be identified and steps taken to rectify faults. Equally, such operational observations are often of greater value to those preparing to plan and build than any in-depth evaluation report. Where light touch evaluation visits have been carried out, it has been found that these are very beneficial, and also reflect a continuing interest with a project once it has become live.

Acknowledgements

Acknowledgements should be made to:

- Cancer Relief Macmillan Fund, London who commissioned the development and design of the Macmillan Green Planning concept.
- Architects Design Partnership, Yeovil who were responsible for the design development of Macmillan Green.
- Northcroft, Quantity Surveyors, Oxford who have managed all the day unit developments in the UK for which Cancer Relief has been responsible.
- May I extend personal thanks to the staff of our Planning Office in Bromsgrove who have helped and supported me with the development of our day unit programmes throughout Britain.

Further reading

Macmillan Green – a new planning concept for the care of cancer patients. London: Cancer Relief Macmillan Fund, 1987.
Macmillan Green – from vision to reality. Hosplan Planning and Design Team in association with Cancer Relief Macmillan Fund, 1992.

O'Reilly JJN. *Better briefing means better buildings.* Building Research Establishment, London: Department of the Environment, 1987.

Spooner DP. A British perspective on hospice. *Amer J Hospice Care* 1986; 24–40.

DOH. *Hospital accommodation for elderly people.* Health Building Note 37 London: Department of Health, 1980.

HMSO. *Buildings for the day care of older people.* Health Facilities Note 02 London, 1994.

HMSO. *Common activity spaces volume 1: example layouts; common components.* Health Building Note 40 London, 1992.

HMSO. *Better by design – Pursuit of excellence in health care buildings.* London: NHS Estates, 1994.

Millard G. *Commissioning hospital buildings.* King Edward's Fund for London, 3rd edn, 1981.

Hospice Information Service. *Setting up and running a day care service (the experience of the St Christopher's Hospice).* London: St Christopher's Hospice.

DOH. *Terminal care.* Report of a Working Group chaired by E Wilkes. DOH Standing Sub-Committee on Cancer, 1980.

Appendix 1: Sample briefing questionnaire for palliative care/hospice services

Completion of this checklist will assist with providing an accurate assessment of operational intent and accommodation requirements. It will also provide a base line for preparation of the schedule of accommodation upon which planning and design can proceed.

	Department/service	Provision proposed	Notes
1	Admission policy		
2	Amenities		
3	Aromatherapy and complementary medicine		
4	Catering services		
5	Computer services		
6	Car parking		
7	Chaplaincy services		
8	Chiropody		
9	Conservatory		
10	Communications		
11	Day care		
12	Dental services		
13	Domiciliary services		
14	Dietetics		
15	Disabled persons		
16	Domestic services		
17	Education programme		
18	Engineering services		
19	Environmental considerations		
20	Estate management		
21	Fire precautions		
22	Furniture and equipment		

23   Grounds
24   Interior decor, art and
     design
25   Laundry services
26   Library services
27   Local authority services
28   Medical gases
29   Medical records
30   Medical services
31   Medical social work
32   Mortuary/viewing
33   Music/television/radio
34   Nursing services
35   Out-patient services
36   Pathology services
37   Pharmacy services
38   Rehabilitation
39   Relatives and staff
     overnight accommodation
40   Residential accommodation
     for patients
41   Security
42   Signposting
43   Smoking policy
44   Staff facilities
45   Staffing
46   Supplies and services
47   Telephone services
48   Transport
49   Visiting policy
50   Voluntary services
51   X-ray services

Appendix 2: Sample activity sheet

Activity space data sheet	*Hospice*: St Michaels
Activity space: Dayroom/activity area: day centre	*Date*: August 1985
Room number:	

Functional design requirements

Facilities needed for the following activities:

Dining area:
1. Patients may be ambulant or with walking aids requiring personal assistance or in wheelchairs to eat and drink.
2. Staff and/or volunteers to prepare for and serve beverages and midday meals (Monday to Friday) to patients seated at dining tables. Table heights require consideration.
3. The dining area may also be used for staff/visitors at weekends or other times when the day centre is not in use for patients.

Activity area:
4. Group and social activities with or without music.
5. Diversional therapy.
6. Individual treatment and re-education of patients in walking and other movements whose treatment may require the use of specialised equipment requiring space for use as well as circulation space.
7. Storage/display for books, magazines, record player, etc.
8. Wall display for selected items, posters and pictures.
9. Creation of focal point; fireplace.
10. Television viewing.
11. Film projection facilities: 95% blackout.
12. Creation of a relaxing, interesting environment.
13. This accommodation may be used for religious services from time to time.
14. Patient/nurse call system.

Design notes: Carpet and wallpaper, handrails as appropriate, creation of 'small patient groups'.
Furniture and equipment: Separate schedule.

Number of personnel
       Dining: 15 places + 6 staff
       Activity area: 10–15 patients + staff/volunteers

Planning relationship:
       As planned

Appendix 3: Draft schedule of accommodation – day unit

Table 6.1 Draft schedule of accommodation – day unit

1.	*The Green*	Approx. area (m²)
	Entrance lobby	3.6
	Activity area	24.2
	Dining area	37.8
	Sitting area	24.2
	Conservatory	59.8
	Chapel	14.4
	Coffee bar	9.3
	Physiotherapy	15.0
	External works	–
2.	*Day care support block*	
	Home care office	17.5
	Activity kitchen	13.6
	Quiet room	9.9
	Home care store	7.6
	Staff WC	3.1
	Assisted WC	5.9
	Assisted shower	7.3
	Assisted bathroom	19.2
	In house store	4.9
	Consultant/treatment	17.0
	Interview room	10.4
	Unit office	10.5
	Sitting area	12.0
	Cleaner	6.3
	Corridor	–
3.	*Small utility block*	
	Wheelchair store	4.0
	Hair salon	11.0
	Utility room	10.0
	Disabled WC	4.6
	Corridor	–
	Physio and occupational therapy store 2	10.25
	Visitors' WC	3.1

Appendix 4: Outline cost statement

Set out in Table 6.2 is a notional cost estimate for a day care hospice built along the Macmillan Green planning concept. The figures indicate the prime elements for a completed project and the costs relate to the fourth quarter of 1994 tendering levels (South of England). These costs do not include for Value Added Tax, design fees and expenses, fees for planning and building regulations, furniture and equipment and associated expenses. These on-costs normally amount to around 30 per cent of the construction costs (the land cost and legal fees are a further expense which will also need to be considered).

The costs are based on traditional 'English' construction, this being concrete foundations, brick walls, tiled roofs, plaster and paint finish internally with carpets and full central heating (wet system) and the normal range of electrical installations. The cost also anticipates a 'traditional' procurement method which is competitive with Bills of Quantity and does not anticipate procurement by other methods (e.g. design and build, management contract, etc).

There follows a statement in Table 6.3 expressing these costs of building in other major currencies. These figures can only be for guidance as many other factors need to be taken into account such as construction methods, specification and planning requirements, taxation and the method and culture of procurement.

Table 6.2 Sample cost statement

	£	£/m^2	%
Substructures assuming normal ground conditions	26 000	75.36	6.27
Superstructure (walls, roof partitions, windows, doors, etc)	93 000	269.57	22.41
Wall, floor and ceiling finishings	33 000	95.65	7.95
Fixed fittings (i.e. those normally installed by the builder)	24 000	69.57	5.78
Services (i.e. heating, plumbing sanitary-ware and electrical installations	150 000	434.78	36.14
External works and drainage	89 000	257.97	21.45
Total:	£415 000	1202.90	100.00

(Prepared by Northcroft, Chartered Quantity Surveyors, Oxford, England)
Nominal floor area for a day unit: 345m^2 (gross floor area).

Table 6.3 Schedule of costs based on straight currency conversion

Currency	Exchange rate	Building cost
Sterling	1	415 000
Ecu	1.2881	534 562
Australia	2.0312	842 948
Austria	17.29	7 175 350
Belgium	50.54	20 974 100
Canada	2.1562	894 823
Denmark	9.6231	3 993 587
France	8.4431	3 503 887
Germany	2.4567	1 019 531
Holland	2.7525	1 142 288
Hong Kong	12.1281	5 033 162
Ireland	1.0218	424 047
Italy (100)	2540.16	1 054 166 400

Table 6.3 (*Continued*)

Currency	Exchange rate	Building cost
Japan (10)	156.56	64 972 400
Norway	10.7122	4 445 563
South Africa	5.5719	2 312 339
Spain	206.08	85 523 200
Sweden	11.7657	4 882 766
Switzerland	2.0766	861 789
USA	1.568	650 720

Note: The building cost excludes the following which are equivalent to around 30% (excluding land and legal costs): Value Added Tax; design fees and expenses; fees for planning and building regulations; furniture and equipment; land cost and associated expenses (e.g. legal costs).

Appendix 5: Sample furniture and equipment schedule

Activity space: Day care support　　　　　　　　　　　*Date*: February 1995
Room: Activity kitchen

Group	Item	Qty	Cost per item (£)	Total (£)	Notes
2	Clock	1	25.00	25.00	
2	Dispenser, paper towel	2		N.C.	
2	Dispenser, soap	2	26.00	52.00	
2	Sack holder, large fire retardant	1	45.00	45.00	
3	Blender, hand-held	1	20.00	20.00	
3	Chair, kitchen	4	35.00	140.00	
3	Can opener	1	10.00	10.00	
3	Coffee maker	1	25.00	25.00	
3	Holder, kitchen roll	1	5.00	5.00	
3	Ice-maker worktop	1	300.00	300.00	
3	Kettle	1	25.00	25.00	
3	Kick step	1	30.00	30.00	
3	Oven, microwave	1	250.00	250.00	
3	Processor, food	1	80.00	80.00	
3	Stool, perching	2	35.00	70.00	
3	Toaster	1	35.00	35.00	
3	Trolley, general purpose	1	155.00	155.00	
4	Dustpan and brush	1	4.00	4.00	
4	Trays	2	8.00	16.00	
	Budget estimate for room			£1287.00	

NB. All budget costs exclude VAT.

7

Restorative gardens

Ronald Fisher

'We want to build a hospice, where do we start?' My reply to that question was: 'get as big a garden as you can, and put your building in the middle of it.' A flippant answer perhaps but sound advice nevertheless.

If at all possible, a palliative care day hospice should have a garden, whether it be a backyard turned into a patio with plant containers and a climber up the wall, or a more mature garden with grass, flower beds, trees and running water.

After all, gardens for the sick are not a new concept. They were to be found in the courtyards of the medieval monasteries, where pilgrims and travellers were welcomed into the hospice to rest or for treatment in the infirmatorium. Here there was peace and tranquillity and they grew plants not only for medicinal purposes but for food and drink.

'Restorative Gardens' was the intriguing title of an editorial that appeared in the *British Medical Journal*.[1] It reported that:

recent research in environmental psychology is now giving encouragement to the call for revival of the old tradition of providing gardens for hospital patients.

Modern hospitals with their long corridors, dreary views, harsh lighting, the clutter of medical equipment are environments that produce anxiety, fear and anger,[2] and by contrast, views of trees, lawns, flowers and water promote healing by reducing tension and fatigue.[3]

Any agent, whether it be a drug or a garden, that restores or revives, that is of emotional help, that is truly restorative should be seriously considered. Ernest Grimshaw, an architect said, 'life is commensurate with the number of beautiful impressions that can be squeezed into it'.

The Department of Health,[4] is now saying that hospitals of the future should be beautiful as well as functional. This applies equally to hospice day centres.

Architects are responding to the challenge by following certain criteria, by creating pleasant and interesting landscaping, by providing easy access to gardens, particularly for those patients in wheelchairs, different areas in which to walk and sit, bird gardens, Japanese water gardens, raised flower beds, and low window-sills so that patients in bed, or in chairs in sitting areas, can see the lawns and flowers instead of just the tops of trees. Day care hospices are smaller and more compact and so it is easier to fulfil all these criteria and more.

'We have to capture as many moments of the patient's day as possible', said Dame Cicely Saunders. One way of doing this is to provide a restorative garden – a garden for all the senses.

Patients find great joy in sitting on a patio, or in the shade of a tree, by a fountain or waterfall listening to running water, or strolling gently by the flower beds. 'Flowers are restful to look at', said Sigmund Freud, 'they have neither emotions nor conflict'.

Birds on the feeding tables, splashing in the bird bath, or darting in and out of the nesting boxes do not detract from the tranquillity; neither do the fish in the pond.

Fragrance of a flower is that flower's generosity to be shared by all, and so a scented garden should be created in a raised bed and in the prevailing breeze. A raised bed enables the scent to be enjoyed and the flowers to be touched by patients who do not have to bend down. Raised flower beds also enable patients to do some gardening themselves.

A greenhouse would be an asset. It is unusual if volunteer gardeners cannot be found.

A herb garden can be strategically placed near the kitchen door to provide the chef with ingredients for savouring the food. And, of course, if the garden is big enough it will be possible to grow fresh vegetables and fruit for the patients.

And finally let us not forget that for those who have faith, there is the great satisfaction of being 'nearer to God's heart in a garden than anywhere else on earth'. A restorative garden helps to restore our kinship with nature and revive and renew health and spirit.

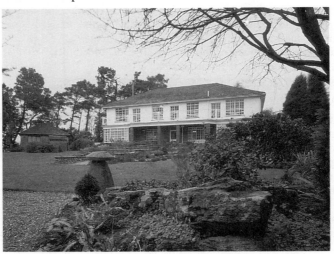

Fig. 7.1 The garden at the Lewis-Manning Day Care Hospice,
Poole, Dorset.

References

1. Warner SB, Baron JH. *BMJ* 1993; **306**: 1080.
2. Malkin J. *Hospital interior architecture*. New York: Van Rostrand Reinhold, 1992; 13–37.
3. Ulrich RS, Parsons R. Influences of passive experiences on individual well being and health. In: Relf D, ed. *The role of horticulture in human being and social development*. Portland, Oregon: Timber Press, 1992; 93–105.
4. Department of Health, *Buildings for the Health Service. London:* HMSO, 1988; (Health Building Note 1).

Part III: Performance

8

Administration and management

David Johnson

Introduction

It would be impossible in a short chapter to attempt a treatise on administration and management (let alone attempt to define the difference between the two!) and to relate this to day hospice services. The last 30 years or so have seen a veritable explosion in management education and management writings. A vast number of management text books offered at varying levels of academic intensity are now available on library shelves. Whilst there is no shortage of practical advice and expertise on how to manage, I think I can best serve the reader by reiterating the core activities of the administration and management function. These are set out in Figure 8.1.

'Miscellany' may strike the reader as a curious description. It is not meant to downgrade the importance of a range of activities (security, data protection, computer development, etc.) which fall within the administrator's remit but merely acknowledges the difficulty of fitting such activities under a 'core activity' heading.

Trusteeship

This section is based on the main duties and responsibilities expected of charity trustees in the United Kingdom. There may be differences in the trustee's role in other countries but the principles of governance and the importance of a clearly understood organisational structure are universally applicable.

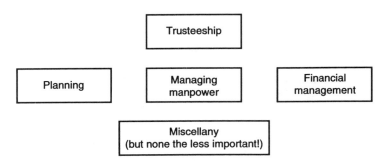

Fig. 8.1 Core activities for the administrative/management function.

In the matter of trusteeship (sometimes called governance) I can do no better than draw the reader's attention to a report on hospice trustees published for 'Help the Hospices' by Trent Palliative Care Centre. The report makes many important points in matters of trustee/management relationships, selection, induction and general organisation. These are summarised below.

Trustee/management relationships

Clear definitions of function should be put in writing, preferably in the form of job descriptions for the chairman, for members of the governing body and for each member of the management team. These will outline what each is responsible for and expected to do and will define scope and limits of delegated powers.

The relationship between the chairman and the management team is a critical one. The chairman's task is to ensure that the trustees support, encourage, challenge and stimulate the management team, without encroaching on their executive responsibilities.

Selection of hospice trustees

Selection of trustees should be based on an agreed assessment of the needs of the hospice and trustees should have personal areas of expertise that fit in with those needs. Job descriptions for trustees should make clear the expected contributions of individual appointees. An indication of time commitment and attendance at meetings is necessary but not in itself sufficient to ensure good corporate governance.

Figure 8.2 shows the responsibilities, roles and requirements of boards of trustees. This helpful model was developed by Stuart Haywood during one of the studies which contributed to the report on hospice trustees.

The induction of trustees

The induction programme for new trustees should aim to provide the same basic knowledge to all trustees at the beginning of their tenure and should include the legal framework, the organisational context and the basic objectives of the hospice. The hospice's mission statement should be given to every new trustee and the induction should be spread over several visits so that relationships can be developed even before the appointment is confirmed.

General organisation

Too large a council of any hospice is to be discouraged. Where the council is large, effective management is likely to be more reliably achieved through small groups or subcommittees of four to eight people working with clearly specified areas of responsibility. These must report to the full council, but can be given wide discretion and power to act between council meetings, subject to ratification. The chairman or other trustees and the management team should formulate an agenda that maximises the contribution of the trustees. This means a selective agenda which should focus attention on items:

1. that require a decision;

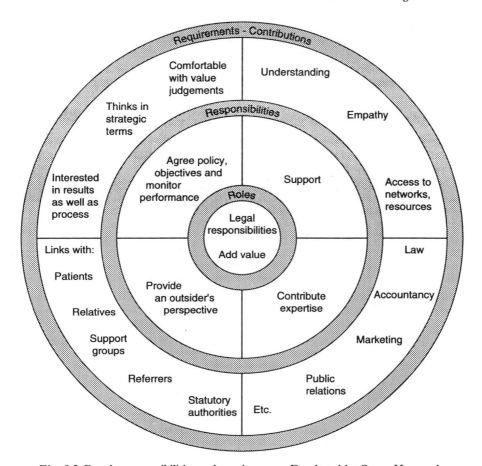

Fig. 8.2 Boards: responsibilities and requirements. Developed by Stuart Haywood.

2. to which the skills of the trustees make a valuable contribution;
3. which are critical to the realisation of targets and developments in business or long-term plans.

Planning

Strategic planning

The planning process is intended to make aims and plans explicit and work out their implications so that a strategy can be developed. The strategy provides the framework for all actions within the hospice. The strategic plan should cover 3–5 years and is merely updated (not rewritten) annually. The exercise must be seen as an opportunity to look critically at different aspects of the hospice's work and future. It must always be seen as much more than the collation of information.

It is important to develop the process only in so far as it helps decision making. There is always the danger that the production of plans becomes an end in itself. The preparation of plans should always be followed by a critical assessment of what has been the value added to decision making and management.

Mission statement

A clear and concise mission statement is the starting point for all planning. It should be directed to purposes and values, not activities. For example (using a fictional name):

> St Paul's Hospice was established to enhance the quality of life of those suffering from cancer and other life threatening illness. It specialises in palliative care and supports those who are in the last phase of their lives, and their families.

This is preferable to stating that it was established 'to provide an integrated palliative care service at Paulsville for its resident population'.

Figure 8.3 is an example of a mission statement. This one was developed for St Mary's Hospice, Birmingham. A good mission statement is not a drafting exercise. It must be *felt* and agreed, and seen to be resolving conflicts, giving clear boundaries to responsibilities.

Mission statement

St Mary's Hospice, respecting the sanctity of life, exists to provide palliative care for those in need, and support for those who care for them.

To this end, we affirm our commitment to:

• Excellence

• Quality of life

• Teamwork

• Education

• Research and development

• Effective use of resources

• Being good employers

• Fairness in our dealings

We believe that good and appropriate palliative care entails the relief of physical, emotional, social and spiritual suffering, whilst respecting the individuality of people and without intention to shorten life.

Fig. 8.3 Mission statement for St Mary's Hospice.

Strategic plans

The content naturally flows from the mission statement and should make clear:

1. Aims in planning period for:
   * development of facilities and equipment
   * each element of the hospice's support operations
   * financial policy, including fund raising
   * organisational arrangements (e.g. more emphasis on marketing)
   * systems (e.g. personnel procedures, quality assurance, contracting).
2. The current situation, including descriptions of:
   (a) need for day care in catchment area of hospice
   (b) current levels of activity provided by the hospice
   (c) services provided by others
   (d) shortfall: a − (b + c)
   (e) views and intentions of referrers and potential purchasers of services
   (f) the organisation:
      * structure (including allocation of responsibilities, lines of accountability and definitions of roles)
      * personnel (type, numbers)
      * volunteers
      * systems (e.g. quality assurance)
      * links with community.
   (g) financial position:
      * trends in spending, income generation
      * financial policies
      * fund-raising strategies and capacity
      * contracts with purchasers, other funds from statutory bodies.
   (h) analysis of hospice operations:
      * strengths?
      * weaknesses?
      * opportunities?
      * threats?
3. Options for development.
4. Choice of strategies for the service and support element. Indications of timing and priority to move from the current situation to achieve the stated aims should be included.

Business plan

The purpose of the business plan is to translate the aims into specific, measurable objectives for the *next* year of the strategic plan. Broadly speaking, they will be of two types:

1. Substantive (e.g. development of amenities, facilities, services, purchase of equipment, appointments);
2. Process (e.g. introduction of quality assurance system, agreements with purchasing authorities, report on case for inpatient facilities).

Note: substantive objectives may include consolidation or maintenance of the current position. For example: 'Numbers of day places will not fall below ...'.

The format of the business plan must reflect local circumstances and preferences. The tests of its usefulness are:

1. Did it improve planning and preparations for the coming year?
2. Is it used to keep a check on progress?

The approach suggested for consideration here is:

3. Summary of targets with timescales and allocations of lead responsibilities backed up by:
4. One page plan for *each* service and facility, and:
5. Each element of the hospice's support operations.

The summary of targets would be the main working document for trustees and senior personnel. The one page plans would be the main working document for those providing the service or support operations.

Managing manpower

A planned, forward-looking approach to the management of expensive human resources requires clear policies on all major aspects of personnel. Policies should:

1. Meet all legal requirements which apply to the employment of staff;
2. Reflect the manner in which the employing authority wishes the service to develop;
3. Form a practical and sensible guide to employment practices.

Some of the areas requiring policy statements are:

- Recruitment
- Retirement
- Equal opportunities
- Health and safety at work
- Discipline and dismissal
- Grievances
- Absence due to injury and ill health.

Given the generally small sizes of hospices, it would be rare to find specialist personnel staff employed. Some larger hospices, however, have introduced staff posts which include a major element of personnel management and the trend appears to be developing.

Recruitment

Before placing an advertisement some important analysis needs to take place:

- Does the job need to be done at all?
- Can it be done by people already employed by the organisation?
- Would the work be better done in a different way?
- What are the financial consequences of the alternatives?

The next stage is to draw up a job description which should accurately reflect the specific job to be done. It may be helpful to separate professional responsibilities and managerial responsibilities and it is becoming increasingly common practice to include a section describing the key result areas.

Once the job description has been completed, the manager can attempt to specify the type of individual who will be required to fulfil the needs of the job description. This part of the exercise – the 'person specification' – is very important and provides an important checklist for the interview.

The next stage is the advertisement itself. The core information allows the reader to know what the job is, the employer, what type of person is being sought, preferred experience and qualifications and a clear idea of the remuneration/benefits of the post.

Shortlisting of applicants for interview should take place against the original 'person specification'. If there is an extremely good response to an advertised post, a good practice is to select a 'long' shortlist (as many as ten or twelve people) and to hold informal interviews before moving to a 'short' shortlist (which should be no more than four or five people).

Once the final shortlist has been settled, the interviews can be arranged. Do not forget at this point to write to referees to give them as long as possible to prepare and submit their references. Key points to observe in the internal process are:

- Clear instructions to candidates as to where the interview is to take place and at what time.
- Indication to candidates as to when the outcome of the interviews will be made known to them. Keeping candidates (successful and unsuccessful) waiting for notification by telephone or by post cannot be regarded as good practice.
- Clear instructions to candidates about what is required of them in the way of 'presentations' at interview and what equipment can be made available (e.g. overhead or slide projectors, flip chart) for visual aids.
- A clear interview plan for the panel at the outset so that it is clear who will be dealing with which area of the 'person specification'.
- Allowing time at the end of the interview for the candidate to ask questions.

When an offer is made to the successful candidate, the contractual relationship between applicant and employer commences. The offer should therefore be made on clear and precise terms and conditions.

Staff appraisal and performance review

'Performance review' is a process to determine how well an individual has performed in relation to the objectives of the organisation. Within these objectives, individuals will have particular aims and targets set for them during the current management year. These will be consonant with the business plan. Performance review is an important aspect of developing individual members of staff and a way of reviewing the effectiveness of a department.

Where staff fail to reach an agreed level of performance, the fault may lie in the target setting. Performance standards must be attainable in the time given if individual grievances are to be avoided. Assistance may be required to enable a member of staff to develop new skills and this should be freely given. Performance assessment and target setting require commitment from both employer and employee.

Health and safety

The Health and Safety at Work Act 1974 provides for an interaction of responsibility for the individuals and organisations associated with work or touched by its immediate consequences. Thus the employer has a duty to his employees with regard to their health and safety and those employees have a duty to one another. The general public are also entitled to a duty of care in terms of safety and health by people carrying out work activities. This includes patients, visitors of all kinds and on-site contractors.

The law imposes a duty on the employer to ensure 'so far as is reasonably practicable' the health, safety and welfare at work of all his employees.

The employer must publish and, as often as may be appropriate, revise a written statement of his general policy with respect to the health and safety at work of his employees and the organisation and arrangements for the time being in force for carrying out that policy.

Matters to be covered in the safety policy include:

- Policy statement and management intention.
- Objectives (in relation to consultation, legal obligations, training, housekeeping, fire, health and hygiene, accidents, etc.).
- Organisation and arrangements.

Financial management

Cash budget (cash flow forecast)

Any business must have money if it is to survive. Remember: many profitable firms fail through lack of liquidity (the ability of an organisation to pay its way). To reduce the likelihood of this happening, a cash-flow forecast or budget should be prepared annually and carefully monitored, if possible on a weekly basis, but certainly once a month.

A typical cash budget working document is shown in Table 8.1. It shows the actual position to the end of December. The rest of the information is based on your best estimate of the likely happenings for the remainder of the financial year.

Budgetary control

Budgeting enables managers to determine levels of service, set standards, agree priorities and compare actual with expected performance. An effective budgetary system encourages better use of resources as well as enabling the hospice to live within income expectations. Budgeting is a way of involving a wide range of managers in economic decisions and should be seen as a helpful discipline rather than a strait-jacket. Budgeting is not just a financial exercise but a means of converting operational plans into action.

Defining the budget content. The expenditure should be structured to reflect the source of decision (for example, signing requisitions, hiring staff). The classification of expenditure headings must be defined and agreed with all managers. The budget should also contain a defined manpower plan for the year in terms of

Table 8.1 St Paul's Hospice Limited: budgeted cash flow to 31 March 1995

	Actual Oct 94 £'000	Actual Nov 94 £'000	Actual Dec 94 £'000	Jan 95 £'000	Feb 95 £'000	Mar 95 £'000
Receipts						
Donations	72	86	98	40	40	40
Covenants	1	1	1	1	1	1
Legacies	54	90	3	10	10	152
Health Authority funding	62	0	286	48	31	49
Interest	0	0	1	0	0	3
Trading profits	0	0	30	30	0	23
Total	189	177	419	129	82	268
Payments						
Salaries	67	67	68	70	70	70
Wages	14	17	15	12	12	15
Inland Revenue	35	33	33	33	33	33
Trade creditors	15	30	21	57	31	31
NHS pension contributions	0	0	0	30	0	0
Other pension contributions	2	5	2	2	2	2
Loan repayment	0	0	0	0	0	53
Total	133	152	139	204	148	204
Opening balance	61	117	142	422	347	281
Movement in month	56	25	280	–75	–66	64
Closing balance	117	142	422	347	281	345

numbers and grades of staff. Manpower plans must be based on planned rotas with an appropriate definition of levels of enhancement, overtime or on-call provision. Budgets should also be set to reflect defined activity levels and service objectives.

The analysis of expenditure. Effective budgetary management requires an analysis which is reliable and pitched at the right level of detail. An effective system of coding will normally define expenditure subjectively by department. The accounts system should be able to consolidate this coding information in several dimensions with appropriate summaries or extracts to meet the needs of managers.

Defining the powers of budget managers. Budget managers are responsible for managing their service within their budgets which should be designed to cover the basic ongoing costs of their departments, taking into account the defined level of service. They should be given flexibility to switch money between expenditure heads within defined parameters.

Flexibility on virement (transfers between budget headings) is also desirable, provided that virement is consistent with budget objectives. Policies on virement and use of savings usually contain check lists on points to be satisfied before virement goes ahead, such as:

- Will appropriate standards be maintained?
- Are budget changes consistent with planning objectives?
- Have the proposals been properly evaluated?

The minimum data set for budgetary control. In order to exercise proper control, budget managers should give attention on a regular basis to:

- Budgeted and actual levels of activity.
- Annual budget analysed by staff grade and type of non-staff expenditure.
- Budget and annual expenditure (or income) for the month, with suitable analysis.
- Budget and annual expenditure (or income) for the period to date with suitable analysis (including commitments where relevant).
- Variance analysis (over- and under-spending, over- and under-income targets) for the period to date.
- The budgeted and actual staffing level by grade and whole-time equivalent.
- *Ad hoc* additional information on problem areas (for example, level of staff absence and turnover).

Miscellany

Computing

When considering introducing computer systems (typically for donor databases, accounting and patient administration systems) first think carefully about what you actually need. You will find it helpful in this process to seek the views of other hospices which have installed computer systems. On the assumption that you wish to proceed, compile checklists for:

- the applications you need;
- assessing the potential supplier(s);
- assessing the software.

Applications: checklist

- For each application list the main transaction types and any files related to these which you currently use. Note current volumes; estimate a factor for expansion.
- Identify any 'non-standard' routines (calculations and unusual constraints within your own current systems).
- Try to identify exceptions which may occur in data passing through the system.
- List all reports you will require with particular attention to their frequency.
- Consider whether you will require any of your applications to run simultaneously.

Supplier(s): checklist

- Tried and tested software used by many organisations is less likely to fail than a new, unproven product.

- Try to buy from a supplier who is likely to remain in business. There is little point in possessing a clever, but unmaintainable, piece of software.
- How long has the supplier been in business?
- Are they helpful and do they have a professional approach?
- Ask for a list of customers and if possible discuss their experiences with them.
- Assess financial stability of the supplier (examine accounts, conduct company search).
- Closely examine terms of sale, paying particular attention to maintenance and support.
- Is any form of training provided or available?
- The location of the supplier also merits careful consideration. Response times can be critical when a system 'goes down'.

With regard to software suitability there are really only two questions to be asked:

1. Will it do the job I want it to do for as long as I need it?
2. How much will it cost?

Software: checklist

- Can the software be customised to meet your requirements?
- Is the system modular to allow expansion?
- What reports can be produced by the systems?
- Is the package well documented and 'user friendly'?
- Are audit trails included to comply with relevant legislation?
- What confidentiality and security facilities are provided including back-up and recovery?
- Can the package be used on other machines within the organisation or must further copies be purchased?
- Can data from this system be shared with other systems or workstations within your work environment?
- Will software be kept in line with changes in legislation?

Data protection

Comments in this section are based on a major area of UK legislation – the Data Protection Act which became law on 12 July 1984. The Act enables the UK to ratify the Council of Europe's 1983 convention for the protection of individuals with regard to automatic processing of personal data and to embrace CECD guidelines on the protection of privacy and trans-border flows of personal data. Since the Act is based upon data protection principles established by the Council of Europe, its parameters will broadly apply to other European countries but readers outside the UK will need to refer to their own country's legislation on this subject.

Purpose of the Act. The Act covers personal data (i.e. data which can be identified as relating to a living individual) held in a form that can be processed automatically (i.e. by equipment in response to instructions given for the purpose). Such personal data and their uses will need to be registered with the Data Protection Registrar and will need to be open to access by the individual on request. Typically in a hospice there will be computer files of donors and employees which will all have to be registered under the Act.

The data user (i.e. the person who controls the content and use of personal data), is responsible for the registration and proper use of the files according to eight principles laid down in the Act. All eight principles apply to a data user.

1. The information to be contained in personal data shall be obtained, and personal data shall be processed, fairly and lawfully.
2. Personal data shall be held only for one or more specified and lawful purposes.
3. Personal data held for any purpose shall not be used or disclosed in any manner incompatible with that purpose (i.e. used or disclosed only in accordance with the data user's register entry).
4. Personal data held for any purpose shall be adequate, relevant and not excessive in relation to that purpose.
5. Personal data shall be accurate and, where necessary, kept up-to-date.
6. Personal data held for any purpose shall not be kept longer than is necessary for the purpose.
7. An individual shall be entitled:
   (a) at reasonable intervals and without undue delay or expense, to be informed by any data user whether he or she holds personal data of which that individual is the subject, and to have access to any such data held by a data user.
   (b) where appropriate, to have such data corrected or erased.
8. Appropriate security measures shall be taken against unauthorised access to, or alteration, disclosure or destruction of personal data.

Failure to comply with the Act can lead to criminal or civil proceedings or both.

Security

Security must be the responsibility of senior managers. It is their job to see that the right policies, procedures and systems are in place and to keep these constantly under review.

The National Association of Health Authorities and Trusts (NAHAT) manual on NHS Security (published in 1992) offers guidance and practical advice on how to draw up an effective security strategy. In addition, a hospice is likely to need expert advice from the police. The provision of security must be balanced so that a deterrent to crime is provided without threatening the comfort of patients or creating a prison-like atmosphere. It must also be integrated with all fire systems so that security and fire arrangements do not conflict.

Security objectives. A security strategy should seek to ensure:

1. the personal safety at all times of patients, staff and visitors;
2. the protection of property against fraud, theft and damage;
3. the smooth and uninterrupted delivery of health care.

Security strategy. Hospices should adopt a formal security strategy. The policy or strategy should set out:

1. the intention of the policy and the management commitment to it;
2. what the policy sets out to prevent;

3. how risks will be assessed;
4. how all staff will be involved in the policy and how particular staff will be given specific security responsibilities;
5. how security fits in with fire arrangements and also with the audit functions of the organisation;
6. where to go for security advice.

Crime prevention. Crime prevention must be the cornerstone of any security strategy. It means anticipating risks and taking action to remove, reduce or transfer them.

Involving all staff. All staff should be involved in crime prevention and security. They should receive induction and annual training covering:

• how best to protect patients;
• how best to guard staff against assault and theft of personal belongings;
• what they are expected to do to safeguard property belonging to patients;
• when and in what circumstances to call the police;
• the scale of the crime problem;
• what management is doing about it.

What can be done to support staff. It is important to do everything possible to protect staff from the danger of assault and to prevent their property from being stolen. Possible ways of doing this include:

• putting adequate security lighting around the premises;
• providing personal attack alarms to staff most at risk;
• providing radio mobile telephone equipment to community staff most at risk;
• installing good quality lockers for clothing and handbags;
• advising staff on the best padlocks for use on personal clothing or handbag lockers.

Complaints

Management should ensure that a complaints procedure is available in the hospice which allows the patient or relatives to seek redress on issues regarding the provisions of the hospice. This should indicate that complaints should be directed in the first instance to the person in charge, and that if the complaint is not satisfactorily resolved it may be referred to the registering Health Authority.

Management will wish to ensure, as a matter of good practice, that complaints are dealt with quickly and effectively and that any justified grievances are promptly remedied.

The duty of the Health Authority in respect of complaints which it may receive is to ensure that there is no breach of the registration requirements, including questions as to the fitness of those working in or responsible for the establishment.

A register of complaints should be maintained in the hospice, detailing the name of the complainant, nature of the complaint and any action taken.

Postscript

As observed in the introduction to this chapter, it is impossible to provide a comprehensive analysis of the administration and management function. To conclude, however, a few 'DOs' and 'DON'Ts' might be helpful.

- DO have a keen awareness of 'season'. By that I mean that the plans, programmes, budget cycle should be firmly fixed in the warp and weft of hospice life and council and committee meetings arranged appropriately.
- DON'T reinvent the wheel. There is a plethora of information available on topics such as employment law, health and safety at work, food handling and hygiene, data protection, security, etc. Consider subscribing to one or more of the organisations that make a business of providing the latest information on such matters but shop around before deciding on your subscription.
- DO remember the hospice movement is still small enough to have very friendly, helpful networks and advice on a problem or even a solution may be just a phone call away. My experience is that hospices are extremely willing to support each other for the good of the movement at large.
- DO have an 'impact' checklist against which all plans and intentions can be judged. This will often be along the lines: 'If we pursued this course of action, then the impact on a,b,c,d, etc. (i.e. the checklist) would be w,x,y,z'.

Further reading

Help the Hospices. *Hospice trustees – the report of a joint working group chaired by A Sayles*. Sheffield: Trent Palliative Care Centre, 1993.

Haywood S, Spurgeon P. *Business plans for hospices*. Birmingham: Health Services Management Centre, 1992.

Health and Safety Executive. *Successful health and safety management*.

National Association of Health Authorities and Trusts. *NHS security manual*. (Working Group chaired by S Shaw). Birmingham: NAHAT, 1992.

9

Community relations and fund raising

Ian Johnson

Some pointers

So your centre needs financial help or maybe the need is to enable you to turn your vision into a reality. Either way, when it comes to fund raising you start with one strong advantage, for particularly throughout the English-speaking world, you are part of a culture in which giving, so often, is very much part of living.

If you have unbounded enthusiasm, strong people skills, limitless energy and move forward in an organised and focused way then the chances are that you will have measurable success. But don't expect that success at every turn – the best laid plans of mice and men . . . .

Let us start from the premise that a group has been formed, charitable status has been obtained and that you have some base to house the organisation. These days there is much unoccupied office accommodation available and it could well be that owners would be willing to let your charity have the space free or for a very limited amount of rent. Try hard to have a location near to the town centre as a real focal point, for it will help raise people's awareness.

One particular point to bear in mind is to let individuals within your group have responsibility for specific aspects of the work. There is nothing worse than 'I thought you were going to do that' and one cannot stress sufficiently the need for clear, planned, and frequent communication within the group. Successes as well as failures need to be shared, for experience gives much added value to the group. Each person must feel involved, appreciated and able to make their personal contribution towards the common goal.

Let us now consider how best you can realise your need – raising funds from your local community.

Public relations

It may sound a little trite, but I have yet to meet the person who contributes to anything without at least some knowledge. Perhaps we should start by first looking at what is meant by the term PR. From the Institute of Public Relations we learn 'Public relations is the planned and sustained effort to establish and maintain goodwill and mutual understanding between an organisation and its public'. Thus PR is very much an ongoing process and not a 'here today, gone tomorrow' concept in the hope that the odd report and article in the local newspapers will solve all your needs.

Firstly, one must be absolutely clear what your message is and to whom it is directed. Long gone – unfortunately – are the days when some well-chosen words in the ears of a wealthy few can magically provide funds completely. The 'old boys' network is still alive but it is unlikely to provide either substantial amounts or, more importantly, continuous support in the years that lie ahead.

What is needed is the wholesale involvement of the community at large; all areas of society who are going to benefit from your centre.

The local media is the first area to concentrate on. Both local radio and newspapers are very much part of the local community. Their raison d'être is essentially to highlight items of interest to local people, and those listeners and readers frequently form a high proportion of the local population including many opinion leaders. There is no better way of communicating with people en masse. You will find that the editorial staff will be interested in your news, your initiatives and the service you provide.

However, do think about your message: precisely what your services are, exactly how the individual can help and what your needs are. A shopping list will not do, so clearly state the real priorities with clarity and conviction. Remember the saying: 'If you try to promote everything, you promote nothing'.

Events

It was not too many years ago that fund-raising events consisted of little more than holding a jumble sale or a coffee morning. I do not denigrate either; in fact over the last 12 months many thousands of pounds have been raised for our hospice by both. However, in the world of events there are a host of other opportunities to raise funds and have fun too. In essence, there are three main methods of fund raising from events. These are:

By selling

For example, people purchasing goods or raffle tickets at a fair, car boot sale (or jumble sale!) or a fete.

By sponsorship

An individual or a team are sponsored for a specific activity. For example a run, a slim, a beard shave, or, in the case of schools, a non-uniform day.

By ticket purchase

This enables someone to be present at a particular function – a dance, fashion show or auction of promises.

Incidentally, there are a number of particular advantages of fund raising from events which frequently result in benefits sometimes larger than the financial result and in addition help other aspects of the cause.

Events will help raise your public profile. Successful involvement with a national or local celebrity will give the media further opportunity to feature local news and a local charity. Secondly, it will provide the means of meeting groups of new people and involving them as contributors and supporters. Finally, the special benefit is to those who work so hard to raise the funds. An event gives the group opportunity to meet with one another, to value each other's commitment and to understand the variety of supportive work done for the common goal. However, one should not underestimate the amount of planning, time and sheer hard work that is often necessary to result in success.

One excellent way to start is to utilise all the expertise, experience and hard work that other people have carried out! Thus it could be that the organisers of a local fete, craft fair or county show would allow you space at their event. That space could be utilised, for example, for a raffle or tombola, selling goods or perhaps just to promote to visitors your services and needs. Is there a local carnival procession in which you could enter a float and collect donations en route? Would it be possible to hold a collection or organise a raffle at a local function?

All these are very real possibilities and it is well worth investing time and a bit of leg work researching libraries and local media to find out what future events and functions are being planned. Who are the organisers? What groups do they represent? How many people have attended in the past? It is important to know as much details as possible before making your approach and that knowledge will enhance your credibility.

The local community is full of enthusiasts. So many people give considerable time to their interests – harness their enthusiasm and ask if they will hold an event in aid of your centre. It may well be that they will need your help not only with the actual event but the pre-event work in selling tickets and publicity. Remember you will be bringing to them the potential of a wider audience (your members) as well as giving them the opportunity of being seen to be supporting a local need.

Involving youth

Ever increasingly, the young are becoming more and more aware of society's needs and involved in making positive contributions. Frequently these contributions are donated to national or international causes and are the result of, for example, a TV programme. However, there is no reason for you to be left out in the cold just because your cause is essentially local. Indeed, it could be maintained that it should be easier for you to achieve success in view of the fact that local people – parents, other relatives and friends – will benefit from your centre.

There needs to be some discussion and thought given as to what you seek from the young. There is considerable difference in motivating a group of teenagers to provide help at a fete and, for example, getting junior school children to fund raise by filling 35 mm film cassettes with coins. Which age group should be your priority? What do you want to achieve? Is it only awareness or some practical help with fund raising? Do you have people who are experienced at working with the young? Talk over your needs and problems with those already involved – head and deputy school teachers, youth community leaders and those who lead Scouts, Guides and other youth groups.

Let me share with you one example of a successful partnership that I was involved in recently. A local primary school had been donating Harvest Festival goods to us for some years and their Parent Teacher Association was looking for new avenues of fund raising to support school funds. After a very positive initial meeting, we agreed to hold a joint 'Auction of Promises'. Before too long we had set a profit target, agreed on a 50/50 split, decided on specific responsibilities with deadlines and things were well under way. More meetings were held and the result of the event was not only a successful social event – with excellent publicity for both of us – but several hundred pounds each to help our respective causes. In addition, I have now worked with and got to know another group – a knowledge which has already proved to be of benefit.

Many local newspapers highlight school and youth groups, who are helping their own development as well as providing support to local charities. A telephone call should soon provide you with details of who their leaders are.

The business community

In spite of the harsh effects of the recession, many companies have continued their policy of providing support to the non-profit sectors. Links with the corporate sector can still prove very worthwhile in a number of ways. Frequently, national companies prefer involvement with national charities, but your particular strength lies in being a local charity, serving local needs and that gives you the opportunity to target largely untapped local companies for their support.

Here is another area where 'homework' needs be done for it is never profitable just to make a 'cold call' with hope in your heart – some time and effort is needed to enable you to stand the chance of success. The 'Big Ask' is never easy but it can be helped considerably by having knowledge of the business and a personal contact. You, your friends, supporters and relations all know people and many of them will be employed by companies in the area. They should soon be able to provide you with up-to-date information, particularly regarding the culture of the company and who's who in personnel. Find out all you can before an approach is made and do have not only specific aims but also clear reasons as to why they should help you. It is also important that you make contact at the right level. In part this will depend on what you are seeking, but the ideal individual will have sufficient responsibility to take decisions and make things happen the way you want. One final point is that a number of companies do have policies which govern their charitable giving and you would benefit from finding out details.

So you now have listed a number of companies and knowledge of both their business and people; how do you make your initial contact? I prefer the personal approach – a telephone call explaining who I am, my role and that I would value a few minutes of their time. Very rarely do I get turned down at this stage and you are now ready for the visit. Business people are busy and it is likely that you will only have a fairly short time to make your case in a positive way.

Explain the service

Explain why the centre is needed, factual information on the numbers of patients helped, and exactly what your service is.

Explain the need

Tell them what the cost is, how the money is to be spent, who have supported you already, and what you want.

How the company could help

Suggest a direct cash donation, a gift in kind (possibly products that they sell), equipment that is surplus, or sponsorship for an event you are planning. Perhaps you could seek staff involvement in getting them to nominate your charity as their charity of the year and hold events to fund raise.

Each year our hospice receives excellent support from a wide variety of local companies – on a few occasions by cash contributions but more frequently by the offer of carrying out a service at subsidised rates or by offering us a wide selection of surplus goods ranging from note paper and filing cabinets to new carpets and office furniture. But the most common form of support we receive is cash from groups of staff who have banded together, perhaps to mark a special occasion, and raised funds to show their support. As so very often in life, one is back to the people and not just the organisation.

Help from the Inland Revenue

All too often national governments change their taxation levels and regulations. It is for that reason that I think it unwise to delve too fully into the various methods by which registered charities can claim back income tax on certain types of financial donations. Briefly, charities can benefit to a very worthwhile degree if financial donations are given under certain schemes:

Deed of covenant

This is a commitment by the donor to an agreed annual donation of a specified amount for a minimum period of 4 years.

Covenanted loan

A one–off donation in place of paying over the minimum period of 4 years.

Gift Aid

A donation, current minimum £250, from either a tax payer or a registered company.

Payroll giving

Donations from an employee over an unspecified period. The amount is deducted by the employer, credited to an official agency, tax reclaimed by the agency and the gross amount sent to the charity.

Collection boxes

Over £50 000 has been raised during the last 5 years by The Friends of our hospice via collection boxes – a magnificent total involving a considerable amount of footwork, coin counting, banking and receipt writing; but all very worthwhile. This amount of money has been raised, in the main, by two methods: namely static boxes out in the community and street/house to house collections.

Static boxes. A volunteer takes responsibility for a particular geographical area.

That person's role is to place in clubs, public houses, shops, work canteens and other public or staff locations as many boxes as is possible for small change donations. Whilst competition is strong, with many other charities' boxes already in place, perseverance can pay off.

Administration is simple, but do keep adequate records of the box numbers, location and date placed. Periodic checks should be made to see if the box needs replacing and it is a good idea to have the telephone number of the volunteer on the box.

Be aware that you will have many surprises! Some locations, thought to be a sure-fire bet, can turn out to be completely disappointing, but the reverse is also true. Undoubtedly, the greater interest you can arouse in the person looking after the box, the better the chances of a high return. So do keep at it, but it is sadly a fact of life that some will inevitably go missing.

Collection days. Licenses to hold a collection day are issued by local councils and many days for next year will already be committed. A well-organised and successful collection day is demanding, with all the organisation concentrated into a short period of fairly hectic activity. A large quantity of people need to be involved, with plenty of reliefs able to take over the work at particular times and all areas with high foot traffic such as bus stations, libraries, taxi ranks and large stores should be fully covered throughout the day. A further need is to ensure that there are sufficient 'runners' to replace full boxes, bringing those filled to one or more central points for ongoing counting and banking.

In conclusion

I would like to underline just one or two aspects of fund raising to conclude.

The development of a quality personal relationship with those who fund raise for your centre is vital. They should always feel rewarded for their efforts and receive a full and detailed letter of thanks. In addition, they should be continually aware of the successes and new needs as things progress.

It is also timely to repeat the need for communication; particularly amongst the leaders of the organisation. They should continually be aware of what has happened, what it is hoped will happen and an all-round knowledge of progress. By doing so, everyone will benefit.

Good luck with your work and every success with your fund raising – and be positive at all times!

Useful addresses

The National Association of Hospice Fund-raisers,
Mrs Carol Walkins (Secretary),
St Francis Hospice, Romford, Essex.
Telephone 01708 763235.

The Institute of Charity Fund-raisers Managers Trust,
Market Towers, 1 Nine Elms Lane,
London, SW8 5NO.
Telephone 0171 627 3436.

Charities Aid Foundation,
48 Pembury Road,
Tonbridge,
Kent.
Telephone 01732 771 333.

The Directory of Social Change,
Radius Works,
Back Lane,
London, NW3 1HL.
Telephone 0171 284 4363.

Professional Fund-raising Magazine,
4 Market Place,
Hertford,
Herts, SG14 1EB.

Charity Magazine,
The Old Court House,
New Road Avenue,
Chatham,
Kent, ME 6BA.

NGO Finance Magazine,
1A Tradescant Road,
London, SW8 1DX.

10

Clinical audit, evaluation and outcomes

Irene Higginson

Introduction

To improve the quality of care for patients and their families several different, but related, approaches have developed. These include clinical audit, evaluation and outcomes, and are described in the following sections. The chapter then describes how clinical audit could be developed in palliative day care. First, however, the chapter considers the reasons why clinical audit, evaluation and outcomes are important.

Why undertake clinical audit and evaluation or measure outcomes?

Improving the quality of the patient's care is a goal of most professionals. This goal can be traced back to 1518, when the Charter of the Royal College of Physicians included: 'to uphold the standards of medicine both for their own honour and public benefit'.[1] Florence Nightingale was one of the first to use outcome measures when she began to routinely assess clinical care by recording whether patients had improved, deteriorated or died.[2] Since then ward rounds, postgraduate lectures and clinical presentations have contributed to the review of medical and nursing performance. However, often these concentrated on individual unusual cases and were not based on explicit criteria for good practice.

Recent pressures to ensure and improve the quality of health care and the quality of life during care have included:

- change in common diseases (and causes of death) from acute (e.g. infectious diseases) to chronic or with a longer time span (e.g. arthritis, heart disease, cancer);
- an increasing population of older people, with far fewer people dying in their youth or middle age;
- change in medical interventions from those which 'cure' to those which are aimed to improve the quality of life, or the quality of dying;
- demand for assessment of interventions to ensure efficacy and cost effectiveness (ensure value for money for the tax payer);
- demand from patients, their families and many professionals for attention to quality of life, rather than just cure (important in many of the drug trials);
- awareness by professionals and drug companies that their products would not affect survival, but quality of life.

Individuals in today's society are much more conscious of their rights to demand high-quality care and, through government, wish to ensure that professionals are accountable for the health care they provide.

Clinical audit

Clinical audit is the systematic critical analysis of the quality of clinical care including the procedures used for diagnosis and treatment, the use of resources and the resulting outcome and quality of life for the patient.[3]

Early forms of audit involved only single professions, such as doctors. However, it is now widely accepted that audit in palliative care should be multi-professional, to reflect the multi-professional nature of care. Clinical audit is like medical and nursing audit but involves all professionals and volunteers, rather than only doctors or nurses.

The audit can be prospective – where the standards and measures are agreed at the start and are recorded on patients and families during their care – or retrospective, which looks back at the care of patients using either the clinical notes and extracting the information or by asking families.

Clinical audit is a cycle where standards or goals are set and compared with reality by observing practice; results are then fed back to improve practice and set new standards, then the audit cycle is repeated. Figure 10.1 shows this cycle. There are variations including ones which show a snowball effect to indicate that the standards and monitoring undertaken evolve as the cycle is repeated. Clinical audit can begin at any point in the cycle, and the cycle varies, but most people choose to begin by either setting standards or by reviewing practice.

There are a variety of other terms for audit (*see* Box 10.1).

Box 10.1 Audit by any other name		
Medical	Care	Evaluation
Health	Standards	Assessment
Clinical	Activity	Assurance
Professional	Review	Audit
Total	Quality	Management
	Monitoring	
Adapted and updated from: Shaw.[4]		

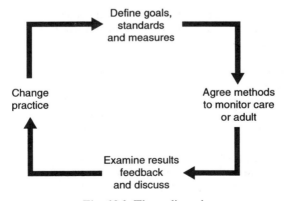

Fig. 10.1 The audit cycle.

Quality assurance and total quality management programmes

Although there are various definitions for quality assurance, a widely accepted one is the 'definition of standards, the measurement of their achievement and the mechanisms to improve performance'.[1] Thus, the cycle is as clinical audit. Clinical audit lies within the frame of quality assurance: clinical audit being the review of the quality of local clinical practice on a regular basis, for example through internal 'peer review' by practising clinicians.

Quality in health care can be seen from various angles: equity and accessibility (the provision and availability of services to everyone in need), effectiveness (achieving the intended benefits within a population), acceptability and humanity (to the consumer and the provider) and efficiency (the avoidance of waste).[1,5] Simple general definitions of quality are available, for example that quality is meeting the customer requirements, or meeting people's healthcare requirements.[6] Of course, quality includes these, but the more comprehensive definitions provide a way of looking at quality in a broad way: the danger of using the simple definitions is that a service may assert it has high quality if a satisfaction survey of patients receiving the service shows it is very acceptable, but the study team have overlooked problems in another area – for example equity or clinical effectiveness.

Total quality management is a term which has recently entered the jargon in quality in health care. It has been defined as a strategy to get an organisation working to its maximum effectiveness and efficiency.[6] It builds on the other definitions, but it switches the focus from quality practised within professionals to the organisation. Thus clinical audit would lie within a total quality management programme. It also introduces the concept of managing the quality process, and using managers to ensure that improvements in quality occur.

Measure for audit and evaluation: structure, process and outcome

Measures of the structure (i.e. the resources, staff), process (the use of resources, e.g. visits, protocols used, drugs used) or the outcomes (results) of care can be used in clinical audit, quality assurance or evaluation (*see* Box 10.2).

Each approach has pros and cons. Outcomes most closely reflect what happens to patients and their families because these look at pain, symptom control and quality of life. However, outcomes are often the most difficult to measure. Process is easier to measure, but is not so closely related to change in a patient's care. It is only valuable as a measure once the elements of process are known to have a clear relationship with the desired changes in health status.

Structure is easiest to measure because its elements are the most stable and identifiable. However, it is an indirect measure of the quality of care and its value depends on the nature of its influence on care. Structure is relevant to quality in that it increases or decreases the probability of a good performance. Further details of the relationship between structure, process and outcome are shown in Box 10.3.

Box 10.2 Structure, process and outcome: in health care[7]

Structure represents the relatively stable characteristics of the providers of care, of the tools and resources they have at their disposal, and the physical and organisational settings in which they work. Structure includes the human, physical, and financial resources needed to provide health care.

Process represents the activities that go on with and between the practitioners and patients. In simpler terms, it is the use of resources. It includes measures of throughput and whether patients were assessed and treated according to agreed quality guidelines, such as treatment protocols. Guidelines are based on the values or ethics of the health profession or society.

Outcome represents the change in a patient's current and future health status that can be attributed to antecedent health care. If a broad definition of health is used, such as the World Health Organization (WHO) definition of total physical, mental and social well-being, then improvements in social and psychological functioning are included. Donabedian included patient attitudes (including satisfaction), health-related knowledge and health-related behaviour within the definition of outcome.[7]

Box 10.3 The relationship between structure, process and outcome

The structural characteristics of care influence the process of care so that its quality can be either diminished or enhanced. Similarly, changes in the process of care, including variations in its quality, will influence the effect of care on health status and outcomes. Thus, there is a functional relationship as follows:

$$\text{structure} \rightarrow \text{process} \rightarrow \text{outcome}$$

Clinical audit and quality assurances can use measures of outcome, process or structure, or a combination of these. Organisational audits tend to concentrate on the organisation, and therefore include the structure and process of care, and not the outcome.

Evaluation and its relationship with audit

In the context of health service, St Leger *et al.* defined evaluations as: 'the critical assessment, on as objective a basis as possible, of the degree to which entire services or their component parts (e.g. diagnostic tests, treatments, caring procedures) fulfil stated goals'.[8] Thus, if audit involves critical, objective assessment of whether the goals of care are achieved, then audit will also evaluate care. Audits of structure would be unlikely to evaluate care, but audits of outcome would.

Why audit palliative day care?

Day care is relatively new in palliative care and has grown rapidly. Although day care only really began to grow in the 1980s,[9] it is now the most rapidly developing service within palliative care.[9] Using data from a questionnaire survey of activity in 1991, Eve and Smith estimated that approximately 4500 different patients attended palliative day care each week, and about 7000 places were available. The number of places varied from four to twenty-five in each centre, and centres might be open between 1 and 5 days per week.[10] The authors suggested that at least two models of day care operated: a medical model and a social model. An observational study which assessed, using a standard format, twelve day care units in England found a wide variation in the policies, types of patients admitted, staffing, activities offered and objectives of day care.[11] Services varied from those that offered mainly social activities to those with a strong medical emphasis. Others provided a mix of these activities. Although some components of day care, for example the arts offered, have been assessed in small descriptive studies,[12] and descriptions of day care are available,[13–15] day care remains largely un-evaluated. A Medline search in February 1994 by the author, for evaluations and audits of palliative or hospice day care published from 1990 to 1994 inclusive, revealed only one study. A questionnaire survey of local general practitioner principals and consultants showed that 13 months after the opening of a hospice in Ayrshire, specialist advice with home care was considered to be the most useful aspect, in-patient beds useful, and day hospice least useful.[16] Clearly, we urgently need to investigate whether day care is a worthwhile investment compared with other forms of support, which of the different models of day care available appear to be most effective and efficient, for which patients and their families and in which circumstances. Comparative evaluation in terms of the effectiveness, appropriateness and costs of day care is needed.

Clinical audit can address these questions only in part, but it could form an important basis for demonstrating whether day care achieves its stated goals or standards, in better defining the medical and social components of day care, and in determining which types of care appear to work best for which types of patients and families.

Steps to audit in palliative day care

The steps to audit have been described in detail in *Clinical audit in palliative care*[17] along with full details of measures already tested in palliative care settings. A summary of the key steps, adapted for palliative day care and including recent developments, is shown below.

Step 1. Plan the audit and sell it to the key people

Before entering the audit cycle some initial investigation and planning is needed. These will form principles for how the audit will run in the future. The mnemonic SPREE may help:

- Start small, cheap and simple and cause a minimum disruption to care.
- Plan. There needs to be a clear plan, which thinks through why the audit might

be important to you. Discuss the audit with relevant staff and colleagues and agree the plan with them.
- **Regular meetings.** Audit meetings, the collection of information and the review of results must occur regularly.
- **Exchange** ideas within the audit group and where possible with other audit groups learning from each other's mistakes and successes.
- **Enjoy.** Perhaps the most important aspect. Audit must be − and be seen to be − educational and relevant to clinical care.

Step 2. Define standards or goals to be monitored

This takes you into the first step in the audit cycle (*see* Figure 10.1). It is usually best to keep it simple, and not try to encompass everything in the first audit. The mnemonic BRAVE sets out the main steps:

- **Borrow** standards, methods and measures from others to save time and resources if at all possible, then adapt these to local circumstances.
- **Reliable** measures or criteria are needed if more than one person will assess the standards, otherwise time will be wasted and the results can mean little.
- **Appropriate** standards and measures are needed, so that staff feel these are truly assessing the work in their setting.
- **Valid** measures and criteria which accurately measure what the investigator sets out to measure is important if audit is to be effective and to achieve the main goal of audit: improving the care for the patient and family. Validity has various components, which are described in detail elsewhere.[18]
- **Easy.** The methods must be simple enough to be understood and to apply in routine practice.

In day care there are various options for measures and standards. One measure which can be borrowed is the Support Team Assessment Schedule (STAS).[13] Details of the measure are shown in Box 10.4. The measure is one of the few which were originally developed for palliative care. It was initially used in home care

---

Box 10.4 Items in the Support Team Assessment Schedule (STAS). Each item is rated 0 (best) − 4 (worst), with definitions for each point.[13]

Nine patient and family items:	*Seven service items:*
Pain control	Practical aid
Symptom control	Financial
Patient anxiety	Wasted time
Family anxiety	Communication from
Patient insight	professionals to
Family insight	patient and family
Spiritual	Communication
Planning	between
Communication between patient and family	professionals
	Professional anxiety
	Advising professionals

and hospital support teams, but is now used more widely. Designed to assess mainly the outcomes of care, it includes aspects concerned with the patients quality of life (e.g. pain, symptoms, anxiety, spiritual and planning needs), the family, communication and the needs of other professionals. To adapt the STAS for palliative day care, McDaid developed and is testing two new items, which more closely reflect the objectives of day care. These items are shown in Box 10.5. Note that these two items have yet to be tested for validity and reliability and are in the development phase. Other palliative measures, such as the Edmonton Symptom Assessment Scale[19] or the Palliative Care Core Standards[20] might also be adapted for day care.

Box 10.5 Items of STAS specifically geared to day care. (Source: McDaid[22])

Sadness/grief
This is how the patient feels about the diagnosis/prognosis (at each recording) and ascertains how they view the present status. The assessment may also reflect the effect of the family sadness on the patient.

0 = No regrets, accepting situation, prepared will, future plans made for family and affairs, mutual acceptance within the family.
1 = Occasional regrets, but facing situation. Living in the present, thinking each day/week is a bonus.
2 = Moderate sadness – lasting for several hours – weeps easily, grieving loss of health, function. Unable to motivate self during these bouts.
3 = Prolonged sadness – up to several days. Concentrations and activities affected. De-motivated – physical symptoms – loss of appetite, anorexic, listless, antisocial, insecurity – fearful.
4 = Overwhelmed by sadness, feels depressed. Unable to concentrate, de-motivated, 'given up' and withdrawn. Physical symptoms as in 3.

Confidence/self worth
This measures how the patient is coping.

0 = Unaffected by illness, able to make decisions, have opinions, feels in control and coping with illness, symptoms and life.
1 = Occasional doubts about own ability to cope, make decisions, have opinions. Unafraid to seek information.
2 = Moderate loss of confidence – fears losing control. Tentative/hesitant to do anything or seek information. Unsure. Feels self conscious.
3 = Marked loss of confidence and self worth. Feels the illness/symptoms dictate the way of life. Not expecting to improve. Physical symptoms exaggerated. Fears seeking information, fears treatment. Marked self consciousness, 'freakish'.
4 = Overwhelmed by fears, physical symptoms, preoccupied, 'given up'. Anxious, isolated, stigmatised, withdraws – mentally and physically. Often stays in bed.

Note: these items follow the general format of STAS definitions – items are scored depending upon the effect of the problem on the patient with 0 usually meaning no problem and 4 being the most severe, usually overwhelming problem.

An alternative approach might be to undertake topic audit,[21] which would concentrate on one topic within day care, and define the measures and assessments for this. Or to devise your own standards, or adapt/add your own items to STAS and test these. Other forms of audit, such as surveys of general practitioners' views, would also be useful.

Step 3. Start to monitor care

Data collection must commence here, and the mnemonic START can help with the stages:

- Set out how the data will be collected – how often, by whom, when.
- Test the system once or twice and make any changes.
- Agree a date to start and end the audit and follow that.
- Reassess how the audit is going in the first few weeks, try and deal with any teething problems.
- Tell everyone how the audit is going, remind them why the audit is happening and make sure new staff know about it.

Step 4. Analyse the results, keep interest in the audit and repeat the cycle

ARISE may assist:

- Analyse often, so that the results are considered early, not when a large amount of data have been collected.
- Review the audit results, the progress of the audit, and the positive and negative effects of the audit on staff and patients to plan the future developments.
- Instigate change – both in working practice and in the audit method used, even if the changes are relatively small, before the audit cycle is repeated.
- Set new standards – to be monitored in a new audit cycle.
- Effect new cycle, building on the results of the previous audit.

Help available

Local

Monies for clinical audit are made available to the purchasers of health care in the National Health Service in England. Therefore, it may well be worth approaching your local health commissioning agency (or health authority) to find out how money for clinical audit is allocated. In most commissioning agencies money is allocated in each financial year. Some agencies examine bids, others make a payment to the health services or trusts and others will agree an audit programme through the contract they hold with the trust to provide health care. Many of the larger health services or trusts, for example a large hospital or community trust, will have appointed audit officers whose role includes assisting clinical staff with audit. Some health services consider this to be an important investment to ensure the quality of care.

Increasingly in the National Health Service commissioning agencies are asking for audit reports as part of their commissioning work. Probably they are most interested in seeing that any problems identified by the audit are being addressed rather than examining in detail the successes and failings. The role of regional health authorities in the UK is changing and many of their responsibilities are being devolved to the district-based health commissioning agencies.

National

There are a wide number of sources of national information on audit and outcome measures. One of the most helpful is the Outcomes Clearing House which is a National Health Service Executive initiative designed to provide information on current work on health outcomes in the UK. The Clearing House encourages any individuals using health outcomes to register on their database. Any person planning a project in this area can then contact the outcomes centre and ask for a search on the database of projects that may be relevant to their own. This is a very good way of contacting people who are already carrying out work with outcomes. The address is shown at the end of the chapter.

In addition we have developed a database of STAS users and a newsletter for the users which can provide information of new developments and adaptations of STAS.

Occasionally, charities of the Department of Health will fund developmental projects of audit or particular projects, so this is worth considering.

Conclusions

Clinical audit, evaluation and studies of outcome are all means to improve the quality of care for patients and families. It is important that this aim is continually kept in mind and that the audit or outcome studies do not become a paper exercise. Palliative day care is insufficiently evaluated at present. Clinical audit and evaluation is needed urgently if day care is to be continued. The chapter has demonstrated that potential measures for day care are available, along with an approach to developing audit.

References

1. Shaw C. *Medical audit. A hospital handbook*. London: King's Fund Centre, 1989.
2. Rosser RM. A history of the development of health indices. In: Smith GT, ed. *Measuring the social benefits of medicine*. London: Office of Health Economics, 1985.
3. Department of Health. Working for patients. *Medical audit: working paper 6*. London: HMSO, 1989.
4. Shaw CD. Aspect of audit. 1. The background. *BMJ* 1980; **280**: 1256–8.
5. Black N. Quality assurance of medical care. *J Public Health Med* 1990; **12(2)**: 97–104.
6. NHS Management Executive. *The quality journey. A guide to total quality management in the NHS*. Leeds: NHS Management Executive, 1993.

7. Donabedian A. The definition of quality and approaches to its assessment. *Explorations in quality assessment and monitoring*. Volume 1. Michigan: Health Administration Press, 1980.

8. St Leger SA, Schneiden H, Walsworth-Bell JP. *Evaluating Health Services' effectiveness*. Milton Keynes: Open University Press, 1992.

9. Higginson I. Palliative care: a review of past changes and future trends. *J Public Health Med* 1993; 15(1): 3–8.

10. Eve A, Smith AM. Palliative care services in Britain and Ireland – update 1991. *Palliat Med* 1994; 8(1): 19–27.

11. Faulkner A, Higginson I, Heulwen E, *et al*. *Hospice day care: A qualitative study*. Sheffield: Help the Hospices, 1993.

12. Higginson I. *Preliminary evaluation of the Chelmsford Hospice Arts Project*. London: Hospice Arts, 1991.

13. Sharma K, Oliver D, Blatchford G, Higginbottom P, Khan V. Medical care in hospice day care. *J Palliat Care* 1993; 9(3): 42–3.

14. Thompson B. Hospice day care. *Am J Hosp Care* 1990; 7(1): 28–30.

15. Petersen S. Beyond hospice care: a survey of community outreach programs. *Am J Hosp Palliat Care* 1992; 9(1): 15–22.

16. Macdonald ET, Macdonald JB. How do local doctors react to a hospice? *Health Bull Edinb* 1992; 50(5): 351–5.

17. Higginson I, ed. *Clinical audit in palliative care*. Oxford: Radcliffe Medical Press, 1993.

18. Higginson I. Clinical audit: getting started, keeping going. In: Higginson I, ed. *Clinical audit in palliative care*. Oxford: Radcliffe Medical Press, 1993; 16–24.

19. Bruera E, MacDonald S. Audit methods: The Edmonton Symptom Assessment System. In: Higginson I, ed. *Clinical audit in palliative care*. Oxford: Radcliffe Medical Press, 1993; 61–77.

20. Hunt J. Audit methods: palliative care core standards. In: Higginson I, ed. *Clinical audit in palliative care*. Oxford: Radcliffe Medical Press, 1993, 78–87.

21. Finlay I. Audit experience: views of a hospice director. In: Higginson I, ed. *Clinical audit in palliative care*. Oxford: Radcliffe Medical Press, 1993, 144–55.

22. McDaid P. New STAS items: sadness/grief and confidence/self worth. *STAS Newsletter*, Webb D, ed. London: Palliative Care Research Group, HSRU, LSHTM, Keppel Street, WC1E 7HT, 1994, 6–7.

11

Education in palliative day care

Jenny Penson

Palliative day care is, of course, a new discipline and, as such, has a growing body of knowledge behind it. The main research has been done on pain control which is arguably easier to measure and evaluate than the control of other physical symptoms, or emotional, social or spiritual ones. Creating this body of knowledge is a complex task, made more difficult by the claim to a philosophy which, in its holistic approach, does not lend itself to scientific research methods. It is not even clear whether palliative care should confine itself to the care of people with cancer, or if it should be applied to a wide range of life-threatening conditions.

However, in most people's minds palliative care is associated with the hospice movement and, therefore, it is expected to provide education on all aspects of care of people with advanced cancer and their families in whatever setting they are cared for. It is likely that as soon as you have opened your doors to your first clients you will receive requests from people who want to visit and learn from you.

Priorities

This can be both encouraging and, perhaps, a little worrying. Initially, there may be the temptation to allow all-comers, for everyone can give a legitimate reason for wanting to visit, and it can be seen as a good public relations exercise to agree. However, an assessment of priorities needs to be made. It may be useful to decide who needs to see the unit in operation and who might be happy to see it either before the clients arrive or after the clients leave. Otherwise, they may feel that they are on show all the time, and while a few might encourage this, and others may not mind unduly, many may mind a great deal but be too polite to say so. Constant visiting is also likely to be at odds with the informal atmosphere that it is intended to create in the day centre.

It can be helpful to find out what the visitor is hoping to gain from the visit and agree some objectives at the start. It then becomes easier to facilitate the experience and to evaluate how worthwhile it has been for the learner. Learners' needs will vary according to their previous experience and the kind of work they do or course they are following. Requests are particularly likely to be received from Pre-Registration Diploma in Nursing ('Project 2000') student nurses and trained nurses on ENB post-basic courses, particularly the 931 and 285 which are the short and long courses on the care of the dying patient and his or her family.

Indeed, many studies have drawn attention to the need for more education for health professionals in palliative care.[1,2,3,4] Therefore, it is not likely to be long before day care staff are asked to give a talk about their work. This may well begin with a request for a description of aims and functions with examples of practice situations.

Here nurses can build on their very broad role in day care. They are involved in pain and symptom control and in some direct physical care, such as changing dressings and assisting with bathing. Rehabilitation will be a feature for some patients. In their counselling role they will be listening to patients' fears and concerns and helping them to find appropriate ways of coping. They are likely to be involved in the application of complementary, diversional and art therapies. She may well be running self-help or even therapeutic groups. Different day centres may provide other services, for example some run a lymphoedema clinic whilst others take groups for holidays.

From this it can be seen that day care can provide a variety of opportunities for learning to very diverse groups of people.

Practice

Education is not only about presenting facts or listening to lectures, it is also about personal growth and this ideal is very much in tune with the humanistic philosophy of palliative care. It is often said that education should inform practice; it is also the case that practice informs education, giving it credibility and, at times, a much needed reminder of reality. Practice and education are two sides of the same coin. There needs to be a commitment to learn, question and evaluate our practice.

The variability in standards of palliative care carried out in general wards was highlighted by the study of Mills, Davies and Macrae (1994)[5] and by Hanks (1994)[6] who points to the need for the philosophy and practice of palliative care to be applied in other settings. Therefore, many see it as a duty to pass on to others their knowledge and skills so that the care of people with advanced illness can be improved, no matter where they live or what services are available to them.

Staff first

We are all teachers and learners and so the starting point for any educational activity is ourselves. Therefore educational opportunities should be made available to all grades of staff in the day centre (including volunteers). This is not only 'in house' education but encouragement and financial support to attend study days and courses and to share with others what has been gained.

This, of course, is primarily about improving patient care, but it is also about valuing everyone in the team. In this way, education can be another way of giving support. It can provide a forum in which practice issues can be discussed and feelings shared, thus encouraging team building which, to be effective, needs to take place on a regular basis. Stress management techniques, assertiveness workshops, self-awareness exercises and team support (as when a 'popular' patient dies), are some examples of education for staff which can be very helpful at appropriate times.

It is also about demonstrating a commitment to education. It is not helpful to expect staff to be involved in teaching others if education is not seen to be valued by their managers.

Philosophy

Education should be incorporated into the written philosophy of the day centre, and into what is sometimes referred to as a mission statement. Ideally this should be at the planning stage, so that it will be part of all strategic planning.

The mission statement will probably affirm that:

- Appropriate opportunities for learning should be available for all staff.
- New members of staff should receive education in the form of a comprehensive orientation programme.
- New information about palliative care should be regularly disseminated to all staff.
- The practice experience of the multi-disciplinary team forms an important educational resource. Provision of books, journals, audio-visual and open-learning materials should be made available to staff and learners.
- Learners need to be treated as individuals and their past experience valued.
- Account needs to be taken of the context in which they work (e.g. independent sector such as hospice, Marie Curie Home, Sue Ryder Home; the National Health Service such as Macmillan Unit, district hospital, community hospital, or primary health care team in an urban or rural community; the private sector such as a residential home, nursing home or nursing agency).
- There needs to be emphasis placed on the application of theory to practice.
- Education should be about an exploration of attitudes and feelings as well as about knowledge and the acquisition of skills. Therefore a variety of teaching methods should be used.
- Education should be planned and objectives set for the learner to achieve.
- Evaluation of these and of the educational process involved should be made.
- A course planning team should be formed to monitor all recognised courses.
- Research activities of all staff and learners should be actively encouraged.

Environment

When educational activities have been incorporated into the ethos of the day centre, it becomes necessary to decide where the more formal aspects are to take place. It may be possible to start by using a room which is not in use all the time or by teaching after patients have gone home. This is, of course, unlikely to be satisfactory for long. It is then that a decision needs to be taken to raise money to convert some other part of the building, or to build an extension.

When planning a new education facility, it is good to think big. The main room needs to give plenty of space and to be informal and welcoming in atmosphere. There needs to be good lighting, and curtains or blinds to windows so that all visual material can be seen clearly. Screens, boards and overhead projection need to be visible from all parts of the room. Likewise, the room needs to be sited away from noise and to have good acoustics. The addition of other rooms which can be utilised for group work when necessary, has to be considered. An office for a tutor needs to be large enough for tutorials to take place comfortably. There needs to be, however small, a library of books and journals and other learning materials which are easily accessible, especially at break-times.

It is essential to have an adequate number of toilets nearby or sessions will often start late due to queues to use these facilities. There needs to be access to space to eat lunch and to make tea and coffee. It can be helpful when facilitating participatory approaches to have tea and coffee facilities in the room where the teaching takes place. A tray, kettle, mugs and provisions in a corner means that the group can stop earlier or later than planned when this seems appropriate. Discussion can be enlivened by being able to relax with hot drinks to hand!

Personnel

It follows that the next question is who in the team is willing to respond to these requests for teaching and what, if any, qualification they already have to enable them to do so. As teaching is considered to be an integral part of the role of the trained nurse, most nurses will have some experience whilst on ENB courses, especially the ENB 998 Teaching and Assessing course. Some may have done the City and Guilds 730 course. All these will have prepared staff adequately to teach as part of their work and to present material to small groups. If there are no staff with experience then it will be necessary to send one on such a course. If there are none with a particular wish to develop this skill, then it may be worthwhile to attract an additional staff member.

Whichever is the case, it needs to be acknowledged that the involvement of staff in education, whether it is by working with those on clinical placements or giving a presentation to a group, can be demanding as well as rewarding. Also, there may be times when education has to take a low priority because of other demands made on staff at busy times or in distressing or challenging practice situations.

When planning to provide teaching sessions it will be helpful to enlist the support of a nurse tutor from the local college who could act, at the least, as a resource or, at the best, as a mentor. If this arrangement can be made it may also lead to more requests for teaching!

So far we have looked at the educational activities of the day centre as being reactive to the demands that are likely to be made on it. However, a decision may need to be taken about the future direction that education may take. It may be time to become proactive and to consider running a regular programme of educational events and, perhaps, some recognised courses.

It is then that the employment of a full-, or even part-time, educational coordinator becomes necessary and the costs of this set against the advantages of raising the profile of the day centre, establishing networks with other institutions, the sharing of expertise and professional concerns, all of which will help to raise the standard of care.

A word of caution here concerning two possible misconceptions. One is that having a member of the team employed as an educationalist will mean that other staff will teach less. On the contrary, it is likely to mean more requests for visiting and teaching and most members of the team will be encouraged to share their areas of expertise on any courses or study days which are run. Therefore, it can increase the workload of the day care team. The other myth is that running such educational activities will raise money for the day centre or palliative care unit. Although there may be some financial gains from these activities, they are unlikely to cover the costs involved.

If a decision is made to develop the educational activities of the day centre, then it may be useful to explore ways of launching the programme. Putting on a multi-disciplinary study day, perhaps inviting some well-known researchers and speakers on palliative care, would raise awareness, provide up-dated knowledge and encourage some participants who would not normally attend study sessions on palliative care. Therefore, it would be important to keep the cost to participants to a minimum. The organisation may decide that, for these important goals to be achieved, it is worth financing it themselves. Another way is to try to obtain some sponsorship from pharmaceutical manufacturers. Another, though somewhat unattractive option, is to make a tiered system of payment for places, so that different grades of staff pay different amounts.

Planning

When planning a comprehensive programme for a year, it may be useful to think of the many groups that could be targeted and, perhaps, place them in order of priority:

1st stage: leaders in the clinical area

• Managers
• Teachers/lecturers.

2nd stage: clinical specialists

• Oncology
• Palliative care: hospice, Macmillan, Marie Curie
• Breast care
• Stoma care
• Hospital-based symptom control.

3rd stage: generalists

• Primary health care team
• Hospital-based staff
• Health professionals from the private sector
• Ancillary staff: health care assistants, home help service.

4th stage: health care learners

• Students of medicine, nursing, social work.

5th stage: other professional groups

• Clergy
• Social services staff
• Physiotherapists
• Occupational therapists.

6th stage: voluntary groups

• Care volunteers
• Driver volunteers

- Cruse
- Samaritans
- Age Concern.

7th stage: other groups

- Teachers
- Police
- Funeral directors.

From this, it can be seen that there is in palliative care what many would consider to be a duty to pass on what has been achieved to as wide a group of health professionals (and volunteers) as possible. Although most would agree that there will always need to be centres of excellence for research in palliative care, in many cases high standards of care can be achieved by generalists who have the knowledge and skills. Therefore, education is vitally important so that people with advanced disease can benefit wherever they live and in whatever environment they are cared for.

At first sight, you may think that mixing these groups together would seem advantageous. After all, the concept of multi-disciplinary education is much valued by educationalists and palliative care has a strong philosophy of multi-professional teamwork. The team is probably wider than in any other specialty and can include chaplains, social workers, physiotherapists, occupational therapists, diversional therapists, complementary practitioners and volunteers. In practice, you may well have found that this usually means bi-disciplinary, that is, a mixture of doctors and nurses.

In attempting to develop bi- or multi-disciplinary education the main aim is to break down barriers between different groups and so enhance communication and respect by fostering an understanding of each other's roles and problems.

However, it is not easy to attract balanced numbers to such a group (cost can sometimes be a factor), or to make the material seem relevant to those with a diversity of needs and perspectives. Linking it with the very different educational contents and methods of existing curricula can also be a difficulty. Incidentally, it is a concept that can put some people off!

Aims

The generalised aims for any education in palliative care, whether it be for a half day study or a short course might include:

- to provide updated knowledge of palliative care;
- to promote the knowledge, attitudes and skills which facilitate effective care for the person with cancer and his or her family;
- to value the experience, expertise and commitment of everyone involved;
- to act as a resource to others.

Methods

The nature of palliative care has not, as yet, been clearly defined and neither have its boundaries. This uncertainty calls for a very flexible teaching style and may be somewhat at odds with the more usual educational methods which tend to be prescriptive.

Methods chosen usually invite much active participation. A relaxed, informal atmosphere is aimed for, where learners can feel able to question and to share difficult practice situations. In this, of course, there is no expectation that a clear-cut answer to a problem may be found. Much encouragement can be gained in sharing uncertainty.

A variety of approaches can be tried and should be mixed when running a whole day or longer. There are many to choose from. For example:

- short lectures
- visiting speakers
- small discussion groups
- workshops
- case study presentations
- topic seminars
- interpersonal skills exercises including role play
- project work
- reflective journals
- problem-based assignments
- learning contracts to link theory to practice
- guided study
- open learning
- supervision of practice
- visits.

In whatever ways education takes place in the day centre, whether via observation visits, mentorship and informal talks or via a planned programme of recognised professional courses and training, Jones *et al.* (1993) conclude 'the challenge for educators is to stimulate and motivate colleagues to practise patient-centred medicine in this difficult and demanding field'.[7] This is the only way to raise the standards of care so that any patient with advanced disease will receive good palliative care wherever they are cared for and whoever is doing the caring.

Herxheimer *et al.* (1985) reminds us that 'It is no slur on the hard work and dedication that already exists to suggest that there is room for improvement'.[8]

References

1. Field D. Formal instruction in United Kingdom medical schools about death and dying. *Med Educat* 1984; **18**: 429–34.
2. Corner J, Wilson-Barnett J. The newly registered nurse and the cancer patient: an educational evaluation. *Int J Nursing Stud* 1992; **29**(2): 170–90.
3. Kelsey S. Can we care to the end? Do nurses have the skills for terminal care? *Prof Nurse* January 1992; 216–19.
4. Doyle D. Education and training in palliative care. *J Palliat Care* 1987; **2**(2): 5–7.
5. Mills M, Davies H, Macrae W. Care of dying patients in hospital. *BMJ* 1994; **309**: 583–6.
6. Hanks GW. Editorial. *Eur J Palliat Care* 1994; **1**(3): 112.

7. Jones RV, Hansford J, Fiske J. Death from cancer at home: the carer's perspective. *BMJ* 1983; **306**: 249–51.
8. Herxheimer A, Begert R, Maclean D *et al.* The short life of a terminal care support team: experience at Charing Cross Hospital. *BMJ* (1985); **290**: 1877–9.

Further reading

Doyle D, Hanks GW, Macdonald N. *Oxford textbook of palliative medicine* Oxford: Oxford University Press, 1993.
Macleod RD, James C. *Teaching palliative care: issues and implications*. Penzance: Patten Press, 1994.
Tiffany R. A core curriculum for a postbasic course in palliative nursing care *Palliat Med* 1990; **4**: 261–70.
Thorpe G. Teaching palliative care to United Kingdom medical students. *Palliat Med* 1991; **5**: 6–11.

12

A holistic view to managing stress

Rita Benor

Empathy, compassion, and love seen to form a literal bond – a resonance or 'glue'
between living things.

Larry Dossey in 'Healing Words'

This chapter will describe the causes of stress and how the management of stress
and its prevention can be incorporated into a day care setting. Patients, their
carers, and professional staff all may benefit through simple yet profoundly effective self-help strategies and complementary therapies. Mechanisms to explain
how these approaches can bring about changes within the body will be explained,
to include the evidence from psychoneuroimmunology in the prevention and
management of illness.

Introduction

Over the last two decades the word 'stress' has become part of everyday language.
Stress cannot be avoided where humans seek to thrive on challenge and ambition,
or where there is a threat to survival. Stress can affect people of any age, race and
environment. It is prevalent throughout the world, and in 1986 it was estimated
that 300 million working days per annum were lost to stress-related conditions.[1]

Stress is not a disease, but a term used to describe a cluster of symptoms. It is
rare that one stress symptom or phenomenon is found in isolation. Stress affects
the individual's physical, psychological, emotional, spiritual and social well-being,
compromising the integrity of the individual's wholeness.

There are many definitions of stress. Originally the term was used in physics to
describe 'the tension or force placed on an object to bend or break it'.[2] The term
may also be applied to the human response, and particularly for the individual in
the palliative phase of illness,

Stress is defined as the disruption of meanings, understanding and smooth functioning
so that harm, loss or challenge is experienced, and sorrow, interpretation, or new skill
acquisition is required.[3]

The stress response

Stress is an integral part of life. Virtually all psychological adaptation that individuals go through has been labelled stress. Stress can serve as a positive as well as a
negative influence. The body responds physiologically to the stimulus and does
not make judgements, but the individual's psychological function can, and this
introduces a way to alter the response and its effects.

Perception and stress

Perception is the individual's unique view on a given situation and the qualitative assessment of a situation. The processing of perception is very complicated. Perception and judgements of what constitutes and evokes a stress reaction are influenced by the following:

- one's overall level of health and well-being;
- the way one thinks about one's self and one's circumstances;
- the meaning one gives to demands;
- the importance placed on caring for one's self and others.

Some individuals have a lower threshold for succumbing to stress, and for creating it by their attitudes and behaviours towards others. In the late 1960s, several stress-related personality variables were explored and personality characteristics were identified.

Type A personality

These people are ambitious in all projects, work long hours, feel indispensable, put themselves under tremendous pressure to meet deadlines (and in doing so often create stress for other people), need to be in control of themselves and others, and over-schedule their time.

Type B personality

These people do not need to strive, to over-prove or over-function. They are less aroused, more complacent with their lives.

Type C personality

These people suppress their emotional needs, are self sacrificing, and prone to develop serious diseases such as cancer and heart disease.[4,5]

CG Jung described further personality variables which are useful in matching the stress management approach to the individual. Jung observed that we are born with a preference for the way we perceive life and its demands:

1. The person with a primary *thinking* function would view the world through logical, linear ways of relating.
2. The person whose primary function is through *feeling* would react to their circumstances through their emotions and feelings, overall a more subjective approach to life.
3. The *intuitive* personality type would be inclined to relate to the world through a sense of inner knowing.
4. The *sensate* personality uses their outer senses in very practical, objective ways to respond to demands and drives.

Everyone has all four aspects in their makeup, but is influenced by their primary function first and foremost.[25]

Clinical relevance

Awareness of these personality types and primary functions facilitates the matching of appropriate stress management methods to individuals' needs and strengths. In Figure 12.1 suggestions are made for techniques which may be relevant to each personality type.

It is important to bear in mind that no one technique is the exclusive answer in a stress management programme. Having a variety of techniques introduces creative and empowering possibilities for patients and their carers, both professional and lay. Using simple, less taxing techniques initially will help the patient to build confidence and discrimination when approaching their stress management programmes. Stress cannot be eliminated from life. The aim is to minimise the potentially damaging and debilitating effects.

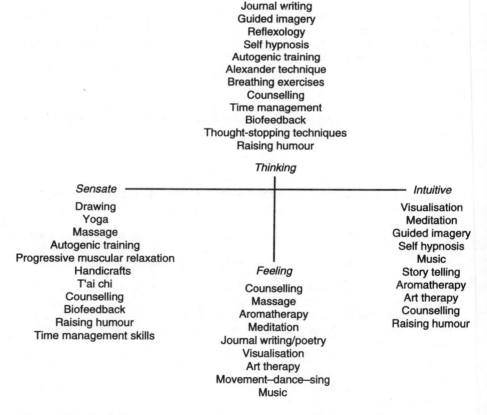

Figure 12.1 Stress management approaches. (Adapted for different primary function from Sharp 1987.[25])

The same personality types and primary functions can be applicable when staffing levels and skill mix are being considered when developing a day care programme and resourcing the staff levels. Much can be gained by having varied and complementary types of personalities working together. This does require that those involved have a tolerance for differences and an openness to sorting them out. The models described are easily understood and can be most helpfully and enjoyably applied to balancing out staffing relationships.

Flight and fight response

When a threat is perceived, it is often accompanied by anger or fear. The stress flight or fight stress response was described by a physiologist, Walter Cannon, in 1914.[6] It has been suggested that the flight and fight response is a basic adaptive mechanism, originally serving to deal with physical threats.[7] Despite increasing psychological sophistication and social advancements, these mechanisms are still the body's way of responding to stress. Hans Selye, an endocrinologist, advanced Cannon's work and described various types of stress. Selye developed his theory to show how physiological reactions operate.[6] The body desires to maintain equilibrium and when a person is aroused through a perceived threat the body reacts to help the person to return to a state of equilibrium and homeostasis. The process is achieved through a serious of complicated neurological and endocrine reactions. Figure 12.2 is a simplified illustration of the neurohormonal stress response.

Cerebal cortex – Limbic system

HYPOTHALAMUS

Corticotrophin releasing factor

Nervous response	*Endocrine response*
Sympathetic nervous system	Anterior lobe pituitary gland
Adrenal gland	Adrenal gland
Medulla	Cortex
Adrenaline/noradrenaline	Glucocorticoids
	Mineralcorticoids

Negative feedback loop

When the stress stimulus has passed, the limbic system reduces the nervous impulse to the hypothalamus, which withdraws the stimulus for adreno corticotrophic hormone (ACTH). The circulating hormones are gradually metabolised and homeostasis is returned to normal.

Figure 12.2 The physiological response to stress.

Types of stress

Selye described three types of stress:

Eustress

This form is associated with pleasurable situations and is termed 'positive stress'. Examples of this may be: the person feels inspired, for instance, to move to a beautiful part of the country to live, to make friends with someone they have admired, to find a new and challenging job, or to plan a good holiday. Essentially, the experience may cause the person to feel an excitement and to be uplifted by it. The pressure or excitement is usually short term and not damaging.

Neustress

This form is stress which is not directly related to the person. The occurrence might be of concern to the individual, but does not directly threaten them. This could include the knowledge that people are starving in Africa, or hearing of a bad road accident on the motorway where one does not know those who were affected.

Distress

This form which is commonly abbreviated to stress, is potentially damaging to the individual.

Stress is subdivided into *acute* and *chronic* stages.

Acute stress is time-limited and is often extremely intense while it is happening. This could be a sudden shock of realising that while you are crossing the road a car speeds towards you with no signs of slowing down, causing you to dash to the safety of the pavement. Other examples might include: anxiety in awaiting a test result, physical injury, or an emotional shock of hearing bad news. Relief is usually predictable.

Chronic stress may also be intense but is more insidious and prolonged, often without any obvious indication of when it will stop. This could, for instance, include the fear of redundancy, a difficult ongoing marital relationship, living with chronic disease or disability, or life-threatening disease with demanding treatment schedules or dependence on medications.

Although the physiological changes are the same for acute stress as for chronic stress, the chronic stress situation sets up a permanent state of arousal. There is an optimal level of stress. When this is exceeded, i.e. eustress shifting to distress, the constant arousal may lead to development of disease and illness, affecting the whole person in mind, body, and spirit. Many diseases are directly related to stress, such as hypertension, diabetes, heart disease, irritable bowel syndrome, cancer, and more.[8]

Burnout

Stress that is overwhelming, cumulative and long term leads to burnout. Burnout is a reaction to too much negative stress and causes the individual to feel totally exhausted, disillusioned, depersonalised and cut off from other people, with reduced performance in all areas of life. In short, a state of total exhaustion is reached.[9] Table 12.1 illustrates the physical, psychoemotional and behavioural changes when stress is prolonged. Table 12.2 describes biochemical response.

Table 12.1 Signs of stress

Physical

Feeling tired and exhausted which is not relieved by rest
Insomnia, shallow sleeping; or disturbed sleep
Headaches becoming frequent and even turning into migraine
Backache
Muscular tension and cramps, particularly in neck and shoulder area
Indigestion, feeling 'butterflies' or knot in solar plexus area
Nausea
Change in appetite, loss/excessive eating/craving certain foods
Changes in bowel habits
Change in menstrual period pattern
Weight loss or gain
Lingering coughs and colds, repeated infections
Slow healing process in wounds
Shortness of breath

Psycho-emotional

Feeling low and moody
Depression
Feeling lacking in motivation
Feeling dispensable
Rationalising
Feeling bored and under stimulated
Restless
Critical of self and others
Feeling criticised (paranoid)
Excessive outbursts of anger, often unprovoked
Crying
Losing their meaning of life
Panic/anxiety attacks

Behavioural

Reduced performance at home or work
Loss of libido or excessive craving for sexual activities
Dependent on stimulants, e.g. coffee, tea, cigarettes, alcohol, food
Repeated sick leave
Unable to take time out

Table 12.2 Responses to stress*

Increased heart rate to pump oxygen to muscles
Increased blood pressure to deliver blood to muscles
Vasodilation of peripheral blood vessels particularly to large muscle groups in arms, neck, back and legs
Increased release of glycogen from liver
Excessive fatty acids released, for sustaining heat and energy
Increased blood coagulation time and a decrease in the clotting time
Muscle strength is increased
Reduced activity in the gastro-intestinal system
Increased perspiration to cool the body
Disturbance to the release of the follicle stimulating and luteinising hormones
Granulation inhibited
Reduced immune response
Reduced inflammatory response

---

*All responses are to provide the body, and in particular muscles, with an opportunity to fly or fight.

Psychoneuroimmunology

Psychoneuroimmunology is the study of the intricate interaction of consciousness, (psycho) brain and central nervous system (neuro) and the body's defence against external infection and internal aberrant cell division (immunology).[10]

There is a vast amount of research in the field of immunology with the subsequent understanding of psychosocial factors and their influence on health.[11] The research evidence suggests that there is a duplication of proteins between the central nervous system and the immune system. This suggests that, in the same way that these proteins carry messages from one nerve cell to another, they carry

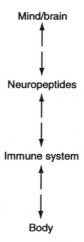

Figure 12.3 Psychoneuroimmunology.

messages from nerve cells to the immune system. The effect is an increase or decrease in the integrity of the immune system and this results in the individual overcoming or succumbing to infection, illness or disease. When combined with the mechanisms of the stress responses, the mind–body connection becomes understandable. Figure 12.3 illustrates this process.

There are a number of studies describing the use of complementary and stress-relieving approaches for patients with cancer. These studies have illustrated significant improvements in the psychological effects as well as improving the immune functioning.[12,13,14,15] In short, if the mental state improves, the physical and immune systems improve.

The fact that people experience stress is not as crucial as how they respond to the stress and how they control it. There are an enormous variety of stress management techniques, all of which may have beneficial effects on the immune system. Some are based on altering consciousness, for instance through relaxation, meditation, hypnosis. Others may be more cognitively based, such as counselling, biofeedback; or may be functional, as with art and music therapy; or may be spiritual, as through prayer, laying on of hands, visualisations and guided imagery. All of these improve the quality of life, enabling the person to take charge of their own care and health maintenance.

For people who have been diagnosed with cancer, the prospects of survival must seem highly uncertain. Living with cancer and knowing that the disease has become chronic and life threatening sets up a situation of chronic stress. This creates a vicious circle of stress predisposing to further stress-induced symptoms, illness and disease. People are often at a loss for anything to do to deal with this constant threat and stress.[16] Unless outside help is offered, people may become severely taxed, further draining their reserves, and exhausting their coping mechanisms. The end result can be that people's overall well-being and quality of life are compromised, resulting in maladaptive physiological and emotional functioning, with diminution of quality of life and worsening of illness and disease. By utilising techniques and interventions which have combined effects on the mind, body and immune system, the person is afforded a better chance of well-being even in the face of pain, unpleasant symptoms, serious illness, and death.

Creating a philosophy for relieving stress

We are all born whole, we have to learn to be unwhole.

Carl Jung

Holistic approaches have a lot to offer when stress management policies of a day centre are being considered. It is frequently inferred that if complementary therapies are involved in care then a holistic approach is taking place. This may not actually be the case. If only the methodologies of complementary therapies are utilised, these may be as insensitive to the individual needs of patients as mechanistically applied traditional medical models.[17]

Complementary therapies are enormously helpful in increasing sensitivity to the patient and in finding ways of reaching into a deeper understanding of their suffering and of their potential self-healing abilities.

Stress management should begin with self care approaches, which empower those who are suffering from the stress to deal with it on their own. This enables them to take their treatment home with them, not relying solely upon the carers exclusively for stress relief. The use of self-healing methods by patients provides a feeling of self sufficiency, a factor often lacking in the presence of illness.

It is essential to apply assessment strategies which explore the individual's needs, taking into consideration their physical, psychological, emotional, social and spiritual deficits and how their illness or stress is interfering with their harmonious functioning.

Whatever the approaches chosen, allowances should be built into the staff schedules for the time these activities will need. While it may seem at first that instructing patients in self-healing methods is time consuming, the opposite is actually the case. These methods are highly cost effective. A single staff member can instruct many patients at once in the use of these techniques. Furthermore, once patients have learned them, they can continue using them on their own.

Assessments should also be ongoing. The faces of stress are many and so often once one area of stress is relieved the person becomes aware of the more subtle layers which have accumulated or which underlie their symptoms. Stress management methods must also take into consideration the levels of functioning in the particular stage of a disease process.

Staff stress and distress can also be addressed through these methods. An open and sympathetic management style can greatly reduce the amount of occupational stress.[18] One of the professional myths of the medical system is that all pain and distressing symptoms can be controlled. This is sadly not the case. This leads to staff frustration for the patient and their family, disillusionment, and exhaustion, resulting in held in emotions which produce chronic stress.[19] In addition, the work environment may not allow the expression of painful or negative feelings. It can be stressful for a patient, their family or staff to have to uphold an implied or expected attitude in dealing with unexpressed thoughts or emotions. The stiff upper lip is slowly being eliminated, but for some it is a coping strategy reluctantly relinquished. How does one complain or just let go when 'everyone is being so nice'?

The notion of the nurse providing full nursing care and also introducing additional skills in complementary care is a wonderful ideal but in reality may not be possible. The blurring of roles can in itself be stressful, where complementary methods have not been included in the job description, where other staff are unfamiliar with the methodologies, and where training and experience of the practitioner are limited. There needs to be full consideration to the conflict of role when one nurse is trained to perform stress-relieving therapies, i.e. relaxation techniques or massage and the like, and is also expected to undertake other generic nursing duties. Policy and procedures need to be thought through about the training requirements the nurse may need before she is competent to provide such additional care.

Stress management awareness for the significant family carer

The effect on the family of someone in the palliative phase of an illness is often an unknown quantity. Bereaved people are at high risk of suffering psychological distress, in the form of anxiety and depression. In addition, often there is impaired the efficiency of the immune system, development of psychosomatic illness and increased risks of morbidity within the first year of bereavement.[20,21,22] More research needs to be undertaken to measure health consequences to the carers during the palliative and terminal phases of illness in order to guide health care professionals and services to prevent morbidity and mortality.

A small-scale study, devised by Marion Garnett, was undertaken to assess the experience of stress due to illness and the desirability of receiving complementary therapies for stress relief in patients and their primary or significant carer. The findings were that both patient and carer had perceivable stress levels and were in favour of receiving complementary therapies. This included the desire for 'talking therapy'. Carers, however, were predisposed to wanting the patient, as a priority, to receive the therapy in favour of themselves.[23] Support groups for carers may facilitate incorporation of self-care strategies amongst carers who otherwise may be reluctant to attend to their own needs.

The day care setting is advantageously placed to monitor the needs of the family. Where practically possible the family or significant carer could benefit from learning stress-reducing strategies. Assessment and awareness-raising questionnaires (as in the Garnett study) would provide information about the day to day pressures on the carer. Stress-relieving techniques could, in themselves, become stressors if consideration has not been given to their integration into everyday demands. Important roles of the day centre staff can include time management and provision of information to aid carers in selecting the most appropriate therapeutic strategy.

The day care centre philosophy and procedural policies of caring for the family carers should reflect support for this extended approach to stress management. There should be sufficient time made available for staff to undertake these assessments. Guidance on the use of self-rated questionnaires would be helpful to provide a basis for designing the assessments around local population needs. It may be helpful as well to have a member of staff identified to implement these policies. Volunteers, trained in stress-management awareness and supervised by staff, could assist in this capacity.

Putting it into practice

Practical considerations must include:

- The provision of an integrated and consistent team of people. Staffing should ideally be of mixed skills.
- Consideration needs to be made towards stress-relieving techniques which will not offend particular religious affiliations.
- Staff could also be supported in attending courses on stress management, humour therapy, storytelling, running support groups, extending their skills so that they become more effective communicators, as well as learning specific techniques and skills.

The British Medical Association and the Royal College of Nursing are exploring the setting of standards for complementary therapies. As with all therapies, however, it is the personality of the person offering the therapy which may be the most healing factor in this process.

Stress release will have to be designed to take into account the level of physical and mental impairment. Conditions such as poor concentration, muscle weakness, reduced or loss of body structure/function, breathlessness and alteration in blood pressure, and effects of medications need to be taken into account when selecting stress-relieving techniques.

Initially the release from stress and tension heightens awareness of just how stressed the individual was. Slow build up from simple to more complex techniques is advisable. Emotional release can initially be upsetting.

Loss of control and helplessness may be typical experiences for people with cancer, with the power for relief and resolution lying outside themselves. People who believe that their health will improve by practising imagery, working to modify and improve relationships, and redefining priorities will typically feel more in control.[24]

The link to all considered here is open mindedness, creativity and effective communication.

> Stress responds to empathy and compassion. Tender loving care (TLC) has uniformly been recognised as an invaluable element in healing pain and distress.
>
> *Larry Dossey in 'Healing Words'*

Four cameo case histories follow, which illustrate actual cases of stress management in palliative care settings.

Case history 1: A man in his early forties was diagnosed with lung cancer

This man had lived a very busy and demanding life and had rarely taken time for himself. He was constantly exposed to stressful work deadlines and family commitments. His prognosis was extremely poor with less than 6 months' life expectancy. He was introduced to and practised daily visualisations, progressive muscle relaxation and received counselling and massage. He lived for another year and expressed his increasing peace and feelings of inner healing, even in the face of approaching death.

Case history 2: Senior nurse in palliative care

I have been nursing for over 15 years and in the hospice movement for 6 years. I was becoming very stressed and feeling that I couldn't keep giving out. I believe I was close to burnout, because I couldn't let go of pent up feelings. I loved nursing but felt unless I found a way of coping I was going to be ill. I was off sick at least once every few weeks. I attended a workshop on stress management and went on to join a weekly meditation group. I feel so much better and have shared some of my simple meditation exercises with a few of my colleagues. It is important to recognise my own frailty not as a weakness but as part of the just being a 'human-being' rather than a human-doing! When facing the death of patients I have come to love and care for, I need care too.

Case history 3: Mother recalling the palliative and terminal phase of her son's illness

My son bravely faced his cancer and its treatment for 2 years. I realised that the time was approaching when the treatment was no longer going to work. My husband and I felt such despair and such helplessness. We were introduced to meditation for ourselves and each day coming together to sit quietly, starting off with prayer, to allow ourselves to find peace in just being in the moment was wonderful. Our son would sometimes join us. He liked it most of all when I gently massaged his body with his favourite aromatherapy oils, or when I led him on an imagery journey. I believe that the stress of our situation, his pain and the subsequent experience of our grief and sorrow was reduced because of what the nurse and other therapists had taught us to do during his dying.

Case history 4: Woman of sixty with terminal phase breast cancer

I have faced many sorrows in my life and after my mastectomy I didn't want to go on. I have found though that there can be profound meaning in illness. I had never been one for talking about myself. I have always been giving to other people, so that when I faced my illness I didn't know how to ask for myself. I have received such help in relieving the stress of leaving my family and invalid husband through counselling, and learning to take time each day to practice my relaxation exercises. My priorities are changed; I can still get anxious and feel panicky, but I now know how to stop and take time to listen to what my worries are. I allow myself to express my anger and I'm no angel, relaxation doesn't award 'sainthood'; what it can do is to help you to understand more about how to let go in a positive way and to let go of worrying for the sake of it. I no longer feel guilty about those things I cannot change. Instead I concentrate on living each day at a time and this has helped my husband and myself to get even closer.

References

1. Cooper C. Survey of stress at work. *J R S Occupat Med* 1986; **36**: 71–9.
2. Seaward BJ. *Managing stress.* London: Jones and Bartlett, 1994.
3. Benner P. *The primary of caring: Stress and coping in health and illness.* California: Addison Wesley, 1989.
4. Simonton O, Matthew-Simonton S, Creighton J. *Getting well again.* London: Bantam Books, 1990.
5. Temoshok LK, *et al.* The relationship of psychosocial factors to prognostic indicators in cutaneous malignant melanoma. *J Psychosomat Res* 1995; **29**: 139–54.
6. Selye H. *The stress of life.* New York: MacGraw-Hill, 1976.
7. Simeons AT. *Man's presumptuous brain.* In: Seaward BJ, ed. *Managing stress.* New York: EP Dutton, 1961; 8.
8. Chopra D. *Quantum healing: exploring the frontiers of mind body medicine.* New York: Bantam Books, 1989.
9. Powell K. *Burnout: what happens when stress gets out of control.* London: Thorsons, 1993.
10. Pelletier K, Herzing D. Psychoneuroimmunology: towards a mindbody model. *Advances* 1989; **5**(1): 27–56.
11. Bauer S. Psychoneuroimmunology and cancer: an integrated review. *J Adv Nurs* 1994; **19**(6): 1 114–20.
12. Fawzy F, *et al.* A structured psychiatric intervention for cancer patients: changes over time in immunological measures. *Arch Gen Psychiat* 1990; **47**: 729–35.
13. Gruber B, Hall N, *et al.* Immune system and psychological changes in

metastatic cancer patients using relaxation and guided imagery: a pilot study. *Scand J Behav Ther.* In: Bauer S Psychoneuroimmunology and cancer: an integrated review. *J. Adv Nurs* 1994; **19**(6): 1114–20.

14. Post-White J. The effects of mental imagery on emotions, immune function and cancer outcome. Doctoral dissertation, University of Minnesota (1991).
15. Spiegel D, Bloom JR, Kraemer HC, Gottheil E. Effect of psychosocial treatment on survival of patients with metastatic breast cancer. *Lancet* 1989; **ii**: 888–91.
16. Gray R, Doan B. Heroic self healing and cancer: clinical issues for the health professions. *J Palliat Care* 1990; **6**: (1) 32–41.
17. Benor R. Holistic nursing: reaching into the foundations of society. *Caduceus* 1994; **24**: 10–13.
18. Hiscox C. Stress and its management. *Nursing Standard* 1991: 5(21): 36–8.
19. Nichols K. Understanding support. *Nursing Standard* 1992; **88**(13).
20. Bartrop R, Luckhurst E, Lazarus L, *et al.* Depressed lymphocyte function after bereavement. *Lancet* 1977; **1**: 834–6.
21. Parkes C. Bereavement. *B J Psychiat* 1985; **146**: 11–17.
22. Schleifer S, *et al.* Suppression of lymphocyte stimulation following bereavement. *J Amer Med Assoc* 1983; **250**: 374–7.
23. Garnett M. Sounding it out. *Nursing Times* 1994; **90**(34): 64–8.
24. Gray R, Doan B. Heroic self healing and cancer. *J Palliat Care* 1990; **6**(1): 32–41.
25. Sharp D. *Personality types.* Canada: Inter City Books, 1987.

Further reading

Davis M, Eshelman E, McKay M. *The relaxation and stress reduction handbook.* Oakland, CA: New Harbinger,1988.

Dossey L. *Healing words: the power of prayer and the practice of medicine.* San Francisco: Harper, 1993.

Gersie A, King N. *Storymaking in education and therapy.* London: Jessica Kingsley, 1992.

Kahn S, Saulo M. *Healing: A nurse's guide to self care and renewal: Yourself.* New York: Delmar, 1994.

Trevelyan J, Booth B. *Complementary medicine for nurses, midwives and health visitors.* London: Macmillan, 1994.

Woodman A. *HEA guide to complementary medicine and therapies.* London: Health Education Authority, 1994.

Part IV: Personnel

13

Staffing in the hospice day centre

Pearl McDaid

Introduction

Each hospice/palliative day care centre has its own style or 'flavour', which has been influenced by a variety of factors. Older buildings which have been converted have an existing ambience, and a 'lived in' feel to them. The newer, purpose built, or even temporary 'make-do' rooms also have an atmosphere. But it is the staff, volunteers, and patients who are going to have the greatest influence on the atmosphere in the day centre.

Throughout the chapters of this book, there is evidence of a common philosophy of care, hope, joy, relief, sharing, enabling, and a love of humanity, at a time when many patients are very vulnerable.

It is necessary that all staff and volunteers should be aware of the philosophy of hospice/palliative day care. The skills and attributes required in a day care leader vary according to the needs of the locality, and the provision of existing palliative care services. Historically, day care was an extension of hospice care, provided for patients who attended from their own homes, with the day centre managed and staffed from the existing bedded hospice ward. In recent years the tendency has been to establish day care in the community, to support the work of specialist and primary health care teams as the next phase in the development of hospice/palliative care services.

The day care leader

This post has been defined in the constitution of the National Association of Hospice/Palliative Day Care Leaders as, 'The person who is responsible for the day-to-day running of the Day Centre'.[1]

The skills, qualifications, and personal attributes required of a day care leader vary according to the needs of the organisation. Generally the person appointed needs to possess organisational, management, and leadership skills. It is cost effective if that person has a health care qualification, for example, either in nursing, or occupational therapy, and who could be employed to utilise these skills in the day centre.

In a newly formed day centre, the day care leader may be required to assist with the commissioning of equipment, and furnishings, and play a key role in the interviewing and appointing of staff members. In many organisations, the day care leader will have a public relations role, and may be expected to assist with fund-raising activities and events.

The day care leader may also be required to assist in formulating the day centre operational policy, and criteria for referral, acceptance, and discharge of patients.

The personal qualities of a day care leader are those that are sought in any employee who works in hospice/palliative care – a mature and well-balanced, optimistic person, whose love of life and humanity is inspiring and motivating. He/she needs to lead and support the day care team in a positive way, but at the same time be able to sensitively facilitate the development of the team dynamics.

The strength and quality of day care is dependent on the personal and professional resources of the team members, and of their working together to create a relaxed and informal atmosphere. It is the day care leader's responsibility to ensure and maintain this ambience, and facilitate the roles of each team member.

The day care team

The demands of the service will determine the size and skill mix of the team. Each team member's role will dovetail with the other, and in some circumstances work in tandem with another team member. The roles are interdependent; therefore, no-one should monopolise the situation, unless it is in their professional remit.[2]

There is undoubtedly the need for nursing skills in the day centre, as many patients require some degree of nursing care, ranging from assisting a patient to have a general bath, to re-siting/re-priming of syringe drivers with diamorphine. Although each day centre has its own operational policy, an increasing number require the senior nurse/sister to assess new patients' needs, and plan, implement, and evaluate programmes of nursing care.

Record keeping

There is an expectation of the day care leader to keep a record of the patient's attendance, and a written report on the care received at each attendance. Most organisations require statistical information that will be used to demonstrate trends, and assist with planning service development.

All staff should be aware of their policy regarding record keeping and of the legal and confidential aspects of patient records.

Drug administration policy

Most day centres have a policy which states that patients attending day care should bring with them sufficient medication as prescribed, for their own needs during the hours of attendance. In general, the patient should be responsible for the safe-keeping and administration of his/her own medication. In certain circumstances, when the patient is judged to be unable to take responsibility for his/her own medication (confused patients), the patient's relative may entrust a nurse member of the day centre staff with the safe-keeping and administration of the medication as prescribed. These medications should be kept in their original container, be clearly labelled with the patient's name and prescribed instructions for administration. They should be stored in a locked cupboard until administered.

The administration of controlled drugs, at the request of the district nurse, (i.e. for re-priming syringe drivers) should be recorded in the District Nursing Notes, which with the exact amount of the drug, should accompany the patient when attending day care.

All the team members should be aware of the requirements of the Health and Safety at Work Act, the fire regulations, the control of substances hazardous to health, (COSHH) as well as their own professional code of practice.

Other services

Bereavement service

Many day centres provide continuing support for bereaved families of patients who have attended day care, especially where there is no formal hospice bereavement support service. Bereavement counselling requires the skills of qualified and experienced counsellors, within a structured framework of support and supervision. However, many day centres find that the families of deceased patients return to thank the staff, and sometimes other patients for the care and companionship afforded to them and their deceased relative.

The day centre may provide a suitable venue for groups of bereaved people to meet in the form of a 'self-help' group or as a venue for a formal bereavement service.

Information service

There is a wealth of leaflets and publications available to anyone seeking information about his/her particular illness, treatments, addresses of self-help groups and advice for carers. Most of the larger oncology or palliative care departments supply written information which is made available to the patients and families.[3]

In areas where written information is limited, it may be helpful to patients and families, if this resource could be provided by the day centre.

Out-patient services

In many day centres where there is a full range of employed professional staff, there is opportunity to develop an out-patient advice and consultation service. In areas where the focus for hospice/palliative care is in a day centre, patients could be referred and attend as out-patients, to receive specific advice from any of the professional staff. It may also be possible for a whole range of treatments to be provided, with or without the full day care service.

These services dovetail into the working pattern of the day centre, but the time allocated for these appointments should be managed carefully. Inevitably, there will be a need for equipped consultation and treatment rooms, and enough staff to assist with treatments.

Advice and treatment from the palliative care doctor at the day centre is a valuable resource to support and complement the primary health care teams, as well as being supportive to the day care team. An increasing number of day centres employ a doctor as part of the multi-disciplinary team, and those day centres which are part of a comprehensive hospice service have allocated 'doctor time'.

Spreading the day care concept

The philosophy of hospice care is known worldwide, and in many countries palliative care is provided in oncological treatment centres. Many of these centres are based in major towns or cities, and it may not be economical or practical to provide the full range of hospice care that is traditional in this country. However, it is possible to provide hospice/palliative care to out-patients by utilising the concept of day care. For those patients who need to travel long distances for consultation or treatments, it provides the opportunity to rest and recover. Thus bringing us to the original definition of 'hospice, a place of rest for travellers'.

Conclusion

Throughout the chapters of this section, the various professionals describe their roles in day care. Most day centres do not have the financial resources that are necessary to fund everyone. However, the utilisation of the skills of volunteers has always been an important and valued part of day care, many of whom are professionally trained, and choose to give their time and energies free of charge.

Although each member of the day care team will be fulfilling his/her own role, the roles will inevitably 'blur'. Each member will be valued for the contribution that he/she makes to the well-being of the patients, and to the rest of the team. The harmony that exists between team members will create the climate that is necessary for accepting the patient as he or she is, and by their attitude, will influence the patient and his/her family towards accepting their situation.

A team that is cohesive, and works well together in a mutually supportive way, will inevitably influence the morale of patients. Laughter in the day centre is a sign of joy and 'normality'. Robert Holden[4] says, 'A burst of happy, spontaneous laughter is one of the most delightful, wholesome and highly prized of all human experiences'. And it is usually the patients who make us laugh!

References

1. Annual Report 1993. National Association of Hospice/Palliative Day Care Leaders. Available from HELP THE HOSPICES, 34–44 Brittania St, London WC1X 9JG.
2. McDaid P. Day care. In: Fisher R, Penson J, eds. *Palliative care for people with cancer*, 2nd edn. London: Arnold, 1995.
3. BACUP Publications on most types of cancer available. 3, Bath Place, Rivington Street, London, EC2A 3JR.
4. Holden R. Introductory chapter. In: Holden R, *Laughter – the best medicine*. London: Thorsons, 1993.

14

Medical staffing in the day centre

Patrick Russell

Introduction

Hospice/palliative day care centres come in a variety of shapes and sizes and to some extent that may determine their medical requirements. From modest enterprises for small groups of patients meeting perhaps in a church hall with a minimum of professional staff, they range through purpose-built centres standing alone, with extensive facilities and a comprehensive staff, to similar centres integrated in larger traditional hospices. From time to time someone asks if there is any need for a doctor in the day centre at all? Although the patients need palliative care, they are still well enough to live at home and therefore are the chief responsibility of their general practitioners and district nurses. True though that is, nevertheless, gaps occur. Much depends on the availability of those doctors and nurses and their aptitude and experience.

Some 45 years ago, an eminent surgeon and teacher at St Thomas' Hospital, Mr 'Pasty' Barret, said to Dame Cicely Saunders in his characteristically robust manner, 'It's the doctors who desert the dying'. Strong words indeed; but I believe they reflect the vulnerability and sense of failure we all feel, faced with the impending death of one of our patients, and often a lack of confidence in how to deal with the difficult symptoms or emotional distress. Certainly as a newly qualified house surgeon at that time, I had received no training or guidance in those matters. Small wonder that we sometimes avoided that bed in the corner of the ward or the difficult home visit. Thanks to Dame Cicely, who went on to found St Christopher's Hospice with a visionary programme of care, study and research, and the consequent growth of the hospice movement, there has been immense progress in the care of the dying, but there remains a long way to go before it will spread uniformly throughout medicine and nursing.

Haines and Booroff's survey in 1986[1] of 196 general practitioners in North West London questioning the problems that they had in looking after patients at home who were terminally ill, and their perceived needs for both training and support services, revealed:

- 32 per cent had problems in controlling pain;
- 45 per cent frequently or always had difficulties in dealing with emotional distress in patients or relatives;
- 20–30 per cent had problems with inadequate support services and communication;
- 4 per cent (approx) felt the need for more training in symptom control and communication with dying patients.

Those findings confirmed a need for specialist support for patients and families, and for those doctors and nurses who carry the main burden of clinical care in the community.

Early days of hospice care saw concentration on better treatment for dying patients in more homely and peaceful surroundings, often at a late stage of the illness. It was soon recognised that patients also had great needs much earlier in their illness when they were still able to live at home. Home care support and Macmillan Nurses were introduced and day care followed.

Hospice care acquired a new aim – *'to enable patients whose illness has progressed beyond the curative phase, and whose expectation of life is thereby shortened, to continue to live at home for as long as possible'*.

The key words are: ENABLE . . . . . . TO LIVE.

At every stage of a life-threatening illness there are needs for clinical acumen and appropriate treatment from doctors. If that need can be met fully by general practitioners at home or ward doctors in hospital, so much the better. If not, then doctors in palliative care services are there to advise and to complement the roles of their colleagues, and occasionally to fill in where shortcomings exist.

The role of the physician in day care

The role of the physician in the day centre is essentially the same as in any other sphere of hospice activity, but with one important advantage. Weekly attendance of at-risk patients for 5–6 hours affords an unusual opportunity for close observation of their progress and anticipation of problems and crises, with consequent early intervention.

Good communication is of the essence – with patients and their families, their general practitioners and district nurses, colleagues in hospital departments, and, not least, with members of the day care team.

We must remind ourselves constantly that general practitioners and district nurses carry the main burden of responsibility and avoid usurping their roles, or in any way undermining their authority. By the same token, the doctor in the day centre is aware of, and sensitive to, the roles of other professionals, and the interdependency of all who work in the day centre.

Someone wisely said that successful palliative care depends on three components:

1. Control of symptoms
2. Creation of a caring environment
3. Provision of time to talk.

Control of symptoms

This is clearly within the purview of day centre doctors, alongside their general practitioner colleagues. Their knowledge and experience of palliative medicine, together with their close contact with patients attending, places them in a strong position to offer suggestions and advice, especially regarding early intervention and change of treatments.

Creation of a caring environment

This function in relation to the day centre calls to mind first the strength of support that patients derive from each other – so called peer group support. One patient told me that she 'only wanted to come to the day centre to meet and talk to other patients. However kind and understanding the staff may be, they have none of them known what it is to struggle with cancer themselves'. The confident and supportive ambience of the centre and its staff gives security without being dominant or intrusive. The prevailing atmosphere of optimism and happiness, even when some patients are very sick, is a constant source of amazement.

The benefit of ongoing observation of emotional and social needs applies equally as much as it does to clinical change and progress. Changes in morale and levels of anxiety, concerns for the family, problems with the activities of daily living, worries about money and sorting out benefits and allowances, are just a few examples of the kind of matters that bear closely on the sense of well-being or suffering, and *exert a powerful influence on the severity of symptoms*. For that reason, they are very much the concern of the clinician.

Provision of time to talk

This should be seen by palliative care staff as nine-tenths listening, and one-tenth talking. Patients frequently harbour considerable ignorance or misunderstanding of their illness, numerous anxieties and fears, and misplaced concerns or unrealistic expectations. That may be due in part to a sequence of unavoidably brief hospital out-patient appointments, often with different doctors, and to the way the overawing effects of hospitals inhibit questions. Or it may be that the general practitioner has not become closely involved on the assumption that the hospital has it in hand. Much may emerge for discussion at formal consultations with the day centre doctor, but very often, as confidence and trust builds up, more will be confided piece-meal to other members of staff, hence the need for good and open communication between team members.

Topics for 'talk' seem endless. Logically they begin with the illness. What is it? What does it mean? Why? Where has it reached? What will happen? What can be done? What hope is there? Am I dying? How long? What will it be like? Who will help and where will I be? Many other subjects arise . . . life past and present, the family hopes and frustrations, sadness – even gardens, horses, and football! All are grist to the mill of holistic care and create trust and confidence. This kind of talk demands openness and honesty, and I am reminded of lines quoted by a clergy friend from a poem by Emily Dickinson

> Tell all the truth but tell it slant,
> Success in circuit lies.
>
> *Emily Dickinson, Complete Poems No. 1*

Medical activities in the day centre

These fall under four headings:

1. Assessment – initial and review.
2. Problems.

3. Liaison – with other doctors.
4. Team support.

Initial assessment

It is likely that the day care sister will have made a preliminary assessment in discussion with whoever made the referral, and perhaps with the patient as well, but it is of great importance that the day care doctor and sister should together have a detailed and careful consultation with the patient and a close relative or carer. The doctor will lead, simply because of the medical content, and the expectations of the patient. It should be open and relaxed, person rather than disease orientated, and conducted if possible in a triangular configuration to draw in the carer. That way we learn more about shared or different anxieties and fears, separate secrets or collusive denial, and whether there are unrealistic expectations. The aim is not to break down defences, but to enable them to face the future together more closely and realistically. The consultation needs to be open and flexible but with an underlying structure.

A review of the illness

Referral forms are not renowned for their information, and access to previous records is often delayed, especially at independent hospices, but it is helpful to discover what the patient appears to know and understand. It is not uncommon when the progress of an illness is slow or intermittent, and after perhaps several years attending busy clinics, for patients to lose sight of what is happening. Thoughtful explanation and discussion is helpful, and in the long run likely to build rather than undermine confidence. Further exploration may extend, step by step over several consultations, and should be taken gently using open questions and never pressed or hurried. Dr Michael Balint's aphorism often quoted at his psychology seminars for general practitioners at the Tavistock Clinic, London, is apposite: 'If you ask questions all you get is answers' – meaning never the real information.

Current problems

Again open questions reveal the main problems, while direct enquiry may be used to complete the picture with regard to vital functions such as appetite, bowels, breathing, sleep and physical energy. Current use of drugs should be listed and their effectiveness noted.

Physical ability

Strength and the ability to cope with the activities of daily living should be gauged. Whether ambulant or restricted, able to wash, dress and use the lavatory unaided, and the extent of normal domestic activities like cooking, cleaning and shopping.

Social

It is helpful to know about the present or former occupation, whether living alone, and in what type of accommodation, whether there are stairs, and how accessible is the lavatory. The level of support from family, neighbours, district and home care nurses, the general practitioner and others needs to be ascertained. A genogram illustrating the family and where they live, together with any other pertinent observations, is always illuminating and valuable.

Morale

As we listen and observe we are able to assess the level of the patient's morale, the extent of anxiety or fear, whether there is apathy or anger, sadness or clinical depression.

Insight

In their book *The Consultation*, Pendleton *et al.*[2] emphasise that no consultation is complete without the patient's 'ideas, concerns and expectations regarding the illness'. They are what matter to the patient and may not coincide with our own, and we may find ourselves confused and at cross-purposes.

Clinical examination

This is important and must not be neglected, but sometimes it may be considerate and justifiable for it to be limited, bearing in mind how much examination the patient may have been subjected to recently elsewhere. It also depends on the information already at our disposal and our need to know.

At the conclusion of the assessment the problems should be enumerated, and where appropriate graded on a scale of 0 to 4 for severity. Trials are continuing to find an acceptable standardised palliative care database to record such information for clinical purposes, and for use in audit. Suitability for day care should be discussed and a programme for further care outlined.

It is helpful to send a summarised report to the general practitioner to establish the purpose and extent of the day centre's involvement.

Review assessments

These are carried out at planned intervals to assess progress and any need for change in treatment or management. Again a report should go to the general practitioner.

As a day centre becomes more established and accepted, its doctor, with knowledge and experience in palliative medicine, can be a useful source of advice for general practitioners and district nurses about patients they are looking after at home, and not necessarily just those coming for day care. Where there is a team of home care support or Macmillan Nurses it is clearly desirable for the day centre to work hand-in-glove with them. In any event a majority of referrals will come from them and it would be sensible to work towards seeing ourselves as members of one team regardless of the constraints of different and sometimes confusing management structures.

Liaison with other doctors

The value of day care for selected patients is well established, but not everyone is convinced or can see that it has serious clinical purpose. Perhaps for some, over-adherence to the medical model obscures the particular significance of the holistic approach in palliative care. Be that as it may it is beholden on doctors exercising palliative care in the day centre to examine critically the clinical content of their work. It is there, but still medical needs pass unregarded or inadequately managed. To be effective we have to be diligent and thoughtful and maintain impeccable communication with our colleagues whose interest in the patient we share. By that means, patients will benefit, and respect for the contribution of the day centre will grow.

What kind of doctor?

It goes without saying that as well as being versed in the skills of palliative medicine, doctors working in day care should be in sympathy with the holistic approach of hospice care. Essentially two kinds of doctor are required:

A physician in regular attendance

He or she should be available from 1 to 2 hours daily to meet the day-to-day medical needs of the centre. Those include planned assessment and review consultations, dealing with other problems as they arise and making a full contribution as a member of an inter-disciplinary team. Circumstances will determine how this doctor is recruited. Commonly she or he will be a general practitioner with a special interest and appropriate experience as well as time set aside for the centre.

Several academic centres have devised extra-mural courses extended over a year and leading to a Diploma in Palliative Medicine. This may be compared with other diplomas traditionally awarded by medical Royal Colleges in the UK and would appear to be a very suitable qualification for doctors fulfilling this role. Women wishing to return part-time to medicine after having children are often highly suited to this work. Hospices or palliative care units within the National Health Service may be different in so far as they will probably have registrars in training posts and part of their work should be assigned to the day centre.

A consultant physician in palliative medicine

This doctor should be available when special advice is needed. Many independent and NHS hospices at present have a medical director who fulfils that role. A new and promising development more in line with the aims of the UK Care in the Community Act 1990 is the creation of a community consultant in palliative medicine based outside hospitals with the remit to advise on palliative care wherever the patient is. It would seem eminently suitable for them to share extended facilities under the same roof with the home care support nurses and the day centre.

The future of day care

Evolution and change has been the hallmark of hospice and palliative care over the past 30 years. With growing numbers of consultants in palliative medicine and expansion of treatment facilities in day centres, the time is right to consider how the role of day care could be enlarged. In this chapter we have already considered the assessment and review of patients attending regularly as a means of influencing their treatment. With additional space and staff it would seem sensible to extend those functions to other patients who could be referred to the consultant as an occasional event for assessment and advice on how to manage their problems at home. In many cases treatment could be given at the day centre, again using it on an occasional basis which many would none the less find very encouraging and supportive. With the agreement of other specialists some patients could be spared the stress of routine out-patient appointments at other busy clinics without severing their connection.

Conclusion

Dame Cicely Saunders has often been heard to say, quoting the dictionary, a hospice is – 'a place of refuge on a journey' – adding that it depends more on people than bricks and mortar. We have seen the fruit of her vision move out from the hospice to care for patients in their homes, and how day care can contribute. Interestingly those changes came about ahead of provisions outlined in the UK NHS Care in the Community Act 1990 which were to:

• enable people to live as normal a life as possible in their own homes;
• provide the right amount of care and support to help people achieve maximum possible independence;
• give people a greater individual say in how they live their lives and the services they need to help them to do so.

An echo surely of the aims of hospice care and the day centre.

References

1. Haines A, Booroff A. Terminal care at home: perspective from general practice. *BMJ* 1986; **292**.
2. Pendleton P, Schofield T, Tate P, Havelock P. The consultation – an approach to learning and teaching. Oxford General Practice Series, 6. Oxford: Oxford Medical Publications, 1984, 41–3.

15

Volunteer support

Marian Longley

Volunteering in the National Health Service has a long and varied tradition. In the 1960s, when more active recruitment of voluntary help began, the main providers of volunteers were such organisations as The Red Cross, The National Association of the League of Friends, The National Old People's Welfare Council (now Age Concern), and the St John Ambulance Brigade, etc.

The hospice movement inherited this tradition and is well known for its use of voluntary help. Perhaps this is on an even larger scale than in many other areas of health care.

The image of the volunteer has changed over the years from what was perhaps seen as groups of wealthy ladies bestowing their time and kindness upon others less fortunate, to present-day volunteers who come from all walks of life, with varying backgrounds. Becoming a volunteer now also attracts people in part-time work, the unemployed and people who have taken early retirement.

In a hospice setting, such people, by giving of their time, energy and talents and by their dedicated involvement, not only complement but enhance the care offered to patients and their families. They help to bring an additional dimension to the care given by the staff, thus providing an extra personal service. They also act as a link between the patient and the outside world.

The use of voluntary help in palliative care is by no means restricted to the UK but extends to countries such as America, Gibraltar, Kenya, Malta and Poland.

The volunteer in the day care unit

In today's palliative care units, whilst importance is still placed on in-patient care, emphasis on day care has increased tremendously, with many benefits emerging for patients attending palliative care day centres.

On entering any day care centre, whether it be open two, three or five days a week, whether the venue be a small 'make-do' room or a large purpose-built unit, an important feature will be the volunteer involvement. Perhaps it will be the volunteer, in the role of receptionist, who first meets the patient on arrival at day care with a cheery 'Shall I take your coat?' or 'Would you like a cup of coffee or a cup of tea?' What an ice breaker and how comforting this can be for a patient who is coming for the first time and unsure of what to expect. In true tradition volunteers do staff tea bars, but the varied talents and enthusiasm of volunteers are put to use in so many other ways. This is not to minimise the role of volunteers in such areas as the tea bar, as so often a patient's or relative's pent-up emotions are released to the person behind the counter. It is therefore so important to have the right person, with the right attitude and sensitivity carrying out this task.

Within the pattern of a typical day care centre, numerous volunteer roles unfold. Firstly, patients usually travel to a day centre and travel home again by a driving scheme which is operated entirely by the use of volunteers. These volunteers are people who are willing to use their own vehicles, are covered by their own insurance, hold a clean driving licence and are reimbursed for their petrol expenses. As in the case of all volunteer roles, careful selection is imperative.

Once the patient has settled in, perhaps following a chat to some of the other patients, it may be appropriate to think of some form of activity. Who is going to play snooker, bridge or dominoes with the patients, who is going to organise a game of bingo or who is going to motivate patients into using their handicraft skills? After consultation with the day care sister or occupational therapist the volunteers so often take on this role and put such special skills as piano playing, flower arranging, etc. to good use. Many patients find hidden talents in later life by the help and encouragement of a volunteer artist or a volunteer pottery teacher. It is rewarding, not only for the patient but also for the relatives, to see the results of their endeavours. Volunteers with skills in beauty care are always in demand and it is relaxing for patients to sit back and have their nails manicured or their hair washed and set. This 'treatment' not only serves a practical function, but also provides individual attention for that patient and is a time when confidences may be shared.

Of course it may be that some patients won't wish to join in with the activities, preferring to sit and look at a magazine, read a book or even just sit. It is therefore so important that volunteers are sensitive to patients' moods and wishes and to accept them as they are at any given time. The volunteer, like the professional carer, needs to be empathic and sensitive.

Pre-luncheon drinks are something eagerly awaited by some day care patients and volunteers wheeling in the drinks trolley are always a welcome sight. Some patients, especially those living alone, do not always have the incentive, the energy or the enthusiasm to cook for themselves so a choice of lunch, served at a table nicely laid out and decorated by the volunteers, is something to look forward to. Add a glass of wine, a chat with fellow patients, together with the attention of the volunteers and nurses who are on hand to meet the patients' needs, and an ordinary meal is turned into a social occasion.

Afternoon tea, prior to the patient going home, and served with home-made cakes (made by a chef or indeed a volunteer), brings the volunteers in touch with the patients again. How much nicer it is for patients to receive individual attention, together with a smile and a kindly word, when being served their afternoon cup of tea.

'Let me help you on with your coat love', from a volunteer, completes the circle and marks the end of another pleasant day care day. Not quite the end of the day for the volunteers though, as washing up and tidying in day care may need to be completed.

It would be a mistake to think it necessary for all day care activities to take place in the day centre itself for many day care days can take the form of a boat trip, a ride to a local beauty spot, or lunch at a welcoming public house. Again, it is the volunteers who usually provide the transport (whether in the form of their own car or driving the unit's mini-bus) and general assistance. Such assistance may cover a multitude of roles from tea making, fetching ice creams, organising a patients' sing along, to sitting quietly and listening to memories such outings may evoke for patients.

It is only natural in an atmosphere of closeness and friendliness that bonds are formed in the day centre and the listening ear of a volunteer is often welcome, whether it be to share feelings about their illness or to share a laugh. Laughter certainly seems to be infectious in a day care unit and often the whole room will be alive by a patient relating a humorous tale. As well as sharing laughter, of course, volunteers do take part in sharing emotional pain with patients and their support in this way is invaluable to both patients and staff.

Bonding in day care may not just be an individual experience, but may be something shared by the group and therefore the death of a patient belonging to that group may be felt considerably by the others. It is sometimes not only the loss of that particular person but this, in turn, can bring about thoughts of their own mortality. At such times volunteers can be involved, with guidance from the nursing staff, in helping the patients as a group or on an individual basis, to talk about that person, to focus on the things they have shared, and the qualities that person brought and to give thanks for the times they had together. Volunteers may also be distressed by the loss of a particular patient and sharing this not only with the voluntary services manager, but with the patients themselves, may prove helpful.

The increasing input and demand for day care volunteer help is constantly growing in our unit where day care attendances have risen from 690 attendances in 1988–89 to 3415 attendances in 1993–94. The projected figure of 4024 for 1994–95 again shows a further increase.

Volunteer sitter/home companion service

One of the fundamental benefits of day care is to give the carer a break. However, for some patients the time comes when even the journey in the car becomes too much and day care is no longer possible. This is when the volunteer sitter/home companion service can be used. Our own service was initially set up with the prime function of providing short periods of respite, say one morning, afternoon or evening a week for the carer. However, with the addition of more specially selected and trained volunteers we have been able to extend this service to also offer companionship to patients living alone. Owing to its success, this service has now become an integral part of the care we offer to community patients and their relatives, where home care may be preferred and appropriate. Part of this success comes from not only giving the carer a much-needed break, but is also due to them having the security of knowing they are leaving their relative with someone equipped with the experience and knowledge to take appropriate action in case of an emergency and someone who has immediate telephone access to help and guidance from the palliative care unit. Again, the selection, training and support of the volunteers is of utmost importance, but obviously these are people with different strengths to offer to patients and their families.

Volunteer bereavement support

Bereavement support for families and friends is a vital part of total care. Such support cannot take away the pain of grieving but it can greatly ease this hurt. Varying forms of support are offered by Hayward House (*see* Figure 15.1).

Each death is discussed at a weekly multi-disciplinary case conference and appropriate support decided upon for families and friends. If the patient has been visited by a Macmillan Nurse, bereavement support will be continued by the nurse. For other families and friends needing support, generally this will be given by one of our trained volunteer bereavement support visitors. If the bereavement is likely to be especially problematical, the support will be given by the bereavement coordinator, the social worker, the senior nurse or the chaplain. If good support is present within the family or friends or from a local support group, a condolence letter is sent after 4 weeks by our medical director to assess the nature of support being received. How well the family and friends are managing, and any needs, can be indicated on an enclosed form and returned in a pre-paid envelope. Such people also are sent a second letter after 3 months enclosing details of local support groups. All relatives or friends (whatever support is being given) are invited to attend a coffee evening or afternoon approximately 6 months after the death. Finally a remembrance/thanksgiving service is held annually where the volunteer bereavement support visitors are on hand to act as stewards and to provide much of the emotional support and comfort needed by relatives and friends.

This is an outline of one form of bereavement service. However, this form may vary in other palliative care units, as will the depth of volunteer involvement.

Carephones

An additional and very worthwhile service provided by trained volunteers for day patients is the installation of carephones into patients' homes. This gives the

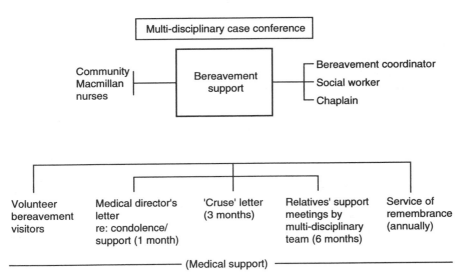

Fig. 15.1 Hayward House Bereavement Support.

patient the reassurance that if they should have a fall or suddenly become ill and unable to reach the telephone, by pressing the emergency button on the pendant around their neck, the telephone will be activated and a recorded message played to one of the telephone numbers programmed into the carephone by the volunteer. Volunteers not only install but check these telephones on a regular basis. This is yet another voluntary service which is increasing, with a growing demand for more trained volunteers.

The voluntary services manager

How does a large band of volunteers, involved in a wide variety of activities, become integrated into a unit's team of carers? Who is responsible for them? Who recruits, trains, places and supports them? This is the role and responsibility of the voluntary services manager (VSM). In the majority of palliative care units around the country VSM posts have become established and unlike the situation of some years ago, in the majority of cases this is a paid post commensurate with the work undertaken.

The role of the VSM may vary somewhat, but the personality of the postholder holds some key factors. When appointing a VSM one is looking for a leader, an organiser, a diplomat, a peacemaker, a juggler of time and resources, and a confidant. Most importantly, a VSM needs to have a sense of humour, be committed and enthusiastic (how else can one hope to motivate volunteers without enthusiasm on the part of the VSM?). The person definitely should not be a clock watcher. If she or he is not willing to give something extra, how can one hope for others to give of their time so freely? The VSM post has its rewards. Along with the volunteers, the VSM reaps great satisfaction from working with the patients and their relatives, colleagues, a committed team of volunteers and from carrying out such a varied and interesting post.

Support for any carer is vital, and it is to be remembered that the VSM may have a large cohort of volunteers to care for at any one time. Who might the VSM turn to for support? The line manager (in my case the medical director) may be the first point of call for both practical and emotional support. Dependent upon the issue of concern, other professional staff in the unit may be willing and able to assist in this way.

On a wider basis, in some areas VSMs have formed their own regional groups which take the form of study days where current topics and related issues may be discussed. These days may also be used as training opportunities for new VSMs in post, as well as ongoing training and up-date for existing VSMs.

Membership of NAVSM (National Association of Voluntary Service Managers), an active association which offers support, guidance and training for VSMs both within the palliative care field and within the general and acute sectors of hospitals, is another means of care available for the carer. The Association of Hospice VSMs was formed especially for VSMs in hospice settings and, again, provides support, guidance and training in the form of regional meetings and national conferences. The VSM may find contact with any of these bodies supportive.

The role of the VSM

So much for the VSM his or herself. Let us now consider his or her actual role within day care. Before even considering recruitment and selection, the VSM, especially if in a new post, needs to lay good foundations for volunteers. If in a National Health Service unit, it is important to know the structure of the palliative care unit and that of the National Health Service on a wider scale. Contacts within the unit, in the Health Service generally, and in the community, are essential, as is a networking system with VSM colleagues.

Close liaison with other members of staff within the unit is so important. Unless properly educated in volunteering, there is a risk they may view volunteers as a waste of time: 'We could be doing the job while we're showing them'; they may be viewed as a threat: 'Is there a risk to my paid post?', etc. As part of my role I endeavour to see each new member of staff during their induction period to allay any fears or scepticisms they may have about volunteers working alongside them. This groundwork is vital for harmonious relations. Staff on all levels need to feel assured that volunteers will be carefully selected, they will have sufficient training before placement, their progress will be monitored and they will be supported by the VSM. If difficulties should arise in respect of a volunteer, staff need to know the VSM will be there to help handle the situation. Staff, therefore, need to have faith in the VSM before we can expect them to accept and have faith in the volunteers.

Recruitment

Before even thinking about recruitment, it is essential the VSM knows the needs of the patients, relatives, the staff and the day centre as a whole. As it is impossible to be in all places at all times to observe all these needs, the VSM must be receptive to the suggestions of others. Consideration needs to be given to the actual task being undertaken by the volunteer. Would it put patients at risk? Would it put the volunteer or others at risk? Are we able to give the volunteer sufficient training for such a task? Will the insurance cover the volunteer and the unit if something goes wrong? It can be a minefield, and unless sufficient thought is given to the task involved and the volunteer's suitability to carry it out, there may be dangers.

Various methods may be used for the actual recruitment of volunteers and recommendation by word of mouth is invariably one of the best forms. Alerting the local volunteer bureau to the needs of the unit may have good results. Inviting staff of such bureaux to the unit for coffee may help them to have a 'feel' of the centre, thereby helping to prevent referral of unsuitable candidates. Publicity in local libraries, health centres, shopping precincts, etc. may also prove fruitful avenues for recruitment. The assistance of the local press may be sought. However, the selection process then needs to be even more carefully undertaken as people may not be applying out of true motivation. Another source of help is the local radio station who may be willing to broadcast an appeal (or allow the VSM to do so.)

Selection

The 'right' volunteer

Selection of the 'right' volunteer is so crucial. It cannot be stressed sufficiently how important it is for time and care to be given to the selection procedure. What qualities might one be looking for to make up that 'right' person?

Obviously where volunteers are required for specific tasks, necessary skills will be important, i.e. handicraft work, driving, etc. However, whatever role the volunteer is being asked to undertake, the most important key feature must be personality. Alongside other features of their make-up such attributes as a mature, sensitive, caring and empathic nature, together with patience, understanding and a sense of humour are essential. Without these basic attributes, whatever training may be given and however much time is spent with a person, they will never become the 'right' sort of volunteer. Drivers may possess years of driving experience, but do they possess the patience, the calmness, the understanding, the caring attitude that are such essential qualities for people who are to be with our patients? Just as nursing professionals will be looking for more qualities in nurses than qualifications, then so must we be looking for such qualities in volunteers. Placing volunteers with patients and their families is a responsibility and should not be undertaken lightly.

The selection procedure

The pathway to selection may take varying forms, i.e. interviewing in the home as opposed to the day centre, the use of a completed application form prior to interview, etc. However, the following procedure is recommended. Upon receipt of a telephone or written enquiry, an information booklet and an application form are sent to the applicant. Upon return of a completed form a mutually suitable date is arranged for interview. All interviews are conducted in the unit, thus giving opportunity for the applicant to see the area where they may be placed and possibly meet patients at all different stages of illness. Ample time should be allowed for the interview, ensuring it is conducted in a room which is free from interruption of people and telephone calls. As with any interview situation, a person may be nervous and unsure of what to expect. This may be helped by such preliminaries as 'Did you manage to park without too much difficulty?', etc. If it appears a person's knowledge of palliative care is limited or their perceptions somewhat misguided, verbally providing some background information may be appropriate. This serves a practical function of information giving, and also provides opportunity for the person to relax and gain composure. This initial meeting should be a two-way process; one whereby information is gained by the VSM about the applicant in order to assess suitability for voluntary work, and one where the applicant gains information in order that they too are in a position to assess if it is what they want and whether they consider themselves suitable for voluntary work in such a specialised setting. There should be no feelings of obligation on either side and complete honesty is essential.

The VSM's prime responsibility is always to the patients and their families but, of course, consideration must also be given to the placement of a volunteer in such a setting.

By the use of skilled interviewing such factors as a person's motivation for wishing to become a volunteer and for choosing such a specialised area, need to be teased out. These reasons may be varied, from 'My GP thinks it would be good for me'; 'My husband thinks I should get out of the house'; to reasons of now having time to do something they have always wanted to do; to give something back in life, etc. Of course, all volunteers need to gain something for themselves by giving of their services and if this is not so, there will be a risk of losing them. However, if the VSM's assessment indicates the applicant's needs are uppermost then the question of suitability needs to be carefully considered. It has to be borne in mind that people with a large amount of instability in their own lives, for whatever reason, i.e. bereavement, illness, divorce, may not have the necessary strengths to offer support to patients and relatives in their time of need. They may also require a disproportionate amount of the support resources.

Some questions will, of course, be hypothetical. A person may not know or may not have given thought to how they would react if present at a death, or how they would react at the sight of unpleasant wounds, but the VSM needs to explore such matters, if only to assess their reaction. The emotional side is another important area which must be explored. Are they the type of person to get too involved? Would they be able to 'switch off' from the patients and the unit when they go home? Would they have sufficient outside interests/hobbies to avoid their voluntary work taking on too high a proportion of their life? This may also be avoided by the VSM ensuring that only a small segment of their time, perhaps one morning or one afternoon per week, is devoted to voluntary work.

Are they able to respect confidentiality? Volunteers may be entrusted with some very personal information and this must, at all times, be kept within the unit. It may be appropriate to ask volunteers to sign against breach of confidentiality. Practical issues will also need to be addressed, i.e. their availability. There may be health issues to be discussed. When interviewing for volunteer drivers it is important to obtain some practical details, i.e. those related to the person's car, how long they have been driving, etc. and it may also be necessary to request a copy of their driving licence and insurance certificate. Knowledge of the person themselves is important; how they would cope with a patient in the car in an emergency, and how they would view a patient becoming unwell in the car with possible temporary damage to the seating. Emergency guidelines should be issued to volunteer drivers but much will also depend upon their personality as to how these are carried out.

If placing volunteers in the day care centre or in-patient area is a responsibility, then it is even more so when placing them in the homes of patients and relatives. In the unit volunteers will have members of the professional team close at hand to help in an emergency but this, of course, is not so in the case of volunteers placed in the community. Although again, emergency guidelines may be issued, so much will depend upon the volunteer remaining calm, in control of the situation and taking appropriate action. It is therefore even more important to select mature, responsible people as volunteer sitters and volunteer bereavement workers. Rather than the VSM interviewing alone, it may be beneficial to draw upon the skills of other professionals to assist in the selection of volunteers for these areas.

The bereaved applicant

It is quite common for relatives and friends whose loved ones have died in the unit, or for those who have had close contact with the day care centre, to offer their services as a volunteer. This may stem from feelings of obligation, of wanting to give something back, or even of feelings of not wanting to lose the attachment that has been built up with the staff of the unit during the course of time. Rather than a mere, 'It is far too soon', over the telephone, it is worthwhile asking the person to come to the unit to talk about this in more detail. Through discussion they may themselves come to acknowledge it is too soon for volunteer involvement. Further contact, after an appropriate length of time, may be offered. This may reinforce the fact that it is the timing that is not right and not necessarily the person themselves.

As with any interview, time should always be allowed for the applicant's questions. Showing a person around the unit, allowing them to meet patients, staff and other volunteers, not only serves a practical purpose, but gives an indication of whether the person feels at ease in the environment, e.g. if they are too shy or too extrovert in their manner when introduced to patients and members of staff.

Armed with sufficient information, together with the knowledge that the applicant is happy to proceed (it may be they would value a short time away from the unit for further thought), the VSM should now be in a position to make an assessment regarding a person's suitability. If all indications point to going ahead then the questions of references and possibly the completion of a health questionnaire need to be raised. In the case of volunteer drivers an appointment for a brief medical may be necessary. Identification badges, showing a current photograph and signature should be issued, especially to volunteers visiting patients' homes. As soon as these formalities have been completed the VSM can go ahead with the next step of suitable training for a volunteer.

Rejection

Rejecting someone is one of the hardest things to do. However, this is very necessary if the VSM knows in his or her heart of hearts that for whatever reason, it would be unwise to accept a person. If it becomes apparent in the early stages of an interview that a person is clearly unsuitable, by the use of skilled interviewing techniques the VSM may change the direction of the interview and pose questions which lead the applicants to realise themselves that this is not the right choice of setting. This self awareness on the part of the applicant is far preferable than an ultimate rejection by the VSM. For the applicant, rejection can be quite demoralising and to alleviate this somewhat, suggestions regarding alternative avenues for voluntary work may be given, i.e. going along to the local volunteer bureau where a whole range of voluntary work may be available. This is a sensitive area and needs to be handled carefully.

Training

Adequate training of volunteers is essential, whatever task they are to carry out. However, it may not be considered necessary for a person helping on the tea bar to be given the same amount of training as a person wishing to undertake work as a bereavement support volunteer. Therefore, the training needs to be matched to the role and should be levelled at equipping the volunteer to carry out the requested tasks. 'General volunteers', i.e. tea bar, flowers, handicrafts, diversional activities, may receive training by being placed with a well-established and experienced volunteer. Volunteer drivers, after a 1-day induction and training course, covering such aspects as lifting and handling, may initially be placed with an experienced driver before undertaking duties on their own.

For volunteers embarking on becoming part of the bereavement or sitter service, special training courses need to be provided. These can be run by the VSM with the help of appropriate professionals from the multi-disciplinary team and outside specialist personnel. Do try to use all available resources, both internally and externally.

Training for such areas as bereavement support and the sitter service may incorporate such practical work as placement, say, for a period of 1 day per week per month, in the day care centre and the ward area. In our own sitter service training, we also incorporate some home visits with a district nurse which gives volunteers opportunity not only to meet patients in their own homes, but also to experience a variety of home settings.

Even though it may not be necessary for every volunteer to undergo a full training course, some form of basic induction is essential for every new recruit. This may cover such topics as philosophy of care, the role of the varying professionals within the centre, policies of the national health service generally and those of the particular unit, etc.

Training should not be considered a one-off event but can be topped up at any time. Ongoing training may take the form of one-to-one sessions or in the more structured form of group sessions. These may be incorporated into support groups or arranged as separate entities.

Placement of volunteers

Day 1 of becoming a volunteer is an important step and it is essential that it runs as smoothly as possible. The responsibility of starting a volunteer should lie with the VSM who at least is a familiar face to the new recruit. Details of the placement, the specific role, etc. are best sorted out prior to the day. It is more than likely that much of the information given when starting will not be absorbed by the volunteer and it is a good idea to have this information typed out, maybe in the form of a small booklet.

What does the volunteer need to know at this stage? Here it may be best to outline some of the major points:

1. Résumé of how the centre is run, members of the professional staff and their role.
2. Policies regarding the overall running of the centre.
3. Policies regarding the remit of the volunteers, their boundaries, etc.
4. A recap of the specific role the volunteer is being asked to undertake.
5. Rules regarding medication, i.e. volunteers are not allowed, on any occasion, to dispense or administer any medication whilst at the centre.
6. Health and safety at work. If there is a health and safety policy relating specifically to volunteers, a copy may be given to the volunteer at this stage. Included in this may be any signing in and signing out policy of the centre, guidelines regarding suitable clothing, wearing name badges, etc.
7. Confidentiality. This is an important aspect, relating to anything they may see, hear or learn.
8. Fire regulations, including the procedure to be adopted should a fire occur whilst they are in the building. Information regarding forthcoming fire lectures.
9. Accident reporting, whether this be to a patient, relative, member of staff or to themselves.

10. General 'do's' and 'don'ts', i.e. policy concerning lifting, handling and toilet-ting patients (whether this is something that must be done by a member of the professional staff only); do not give out home telephone numbers to patients; do not accept monetary rewards; do not offer advice, but do ask a member of the professional team if help is required in any situation. It may be that general talk with a patient can progress to medical matters which a volunteer may not be able – and should not attempt – to handle, in which case they should ask for professional assistance.
11. The unit's responsibility to them – training, support, care and guidance. The unit should ensure that they claim appropriate travel and meal expenses and take regular tea and coffee breaks; and that they are placed in a satisfactory working environment.

See Health Service Guidelines *Voluntary Work in Hospitals* (1992). HG (92) 15.

This is quite an extensive list and a time-consuming exercise. However, time spent at this stage on this ground work (as in the selection procedure) can help to avoid problems at a later date.

Support

Although we are basically placing mature, responsible and reliable volunteers who are able to undertake tasks with the minimum of supervision, continual support for them is essential. This may be merely in the form of saying, 'Thank you, we do appreciate all your hard work', or by lending a listening ear about a particular problem. It may be that on occasion they may wish to discuss something that has taken place within day care or other areas of the unit, which has affected them in some way. Far better this is shared with either the VSM or a member of the staff before they leave, rather than it growing and becoming a problem.

More structured support may take the form of regular volunteer meetings. These may be used also as a means of up-dating volunteers regarding the happen-ing in the unit, further training or an annual fire drill. On occasions volunteers may welcome the chance of getting together for a social evening.

Although volunteers belonging to the sitter service and the bereavement service may welcome the informal support of 'get-togethers', support in these areas needs to be on a more frequent and structured basis. This may be done by offering the facility of one-to-one meetings with the VSM and support groups, held on a regular basis. These groups enable volunteers to meet not only with the VSM and members of the professional team, but also to share their experiences with other volunteers. Immediate contact with the VSM, medical director, senior nurse or social worker can be made if an urgent problem arises, either directly or by tele-phone.

As is apparent from this chapter, volunteering needs to be a structured process if volunteers are to be accepted and integrated into the caring team. Input into the voluntary services is time consuming, not only for the VSM but for other members of the professional staff. However, the benefits to the patients, their relatives, the staff and a unit as a whole are manifold.

Without the volunteers so many of the services which we have now come to take for granted would not even exist.

There is no doubt volunteers reap their own rewards, in turn gaining from the benefits and pleasures they bring to patients, from the social contact and friendship with other volunteers and staff and from the valuable feeling of being part of a worthwhile and dedicated team.

However, I am sure all members of palliative care/hospice teams would agree that these rewards are more than justly deserved, for without the valuable contribution of volunteers, many units would not be the thriving establishments we see today.

16

The chaplain

Bruce Driver

An infiltrator's view

The thing about being a Christian priest is that you never quite belong. You are welcomed into people's lives and the places where they live them. They then often relax and feel comfortable; some of course react quite differently and the atmosphere fills with question marks and anxiety. Either way a priest's presence is always something of a surprise, an ambiguous extra to the regulars gathered at workbench, school, ward, or day centre.

Five minutes on any hospital ward, or in a palliative day care unit, shows us that the priest's inner experience is a kind of focus in illustrating the feeling of not quite belonging which patients, priests, and no doubt God, share.

A seasoned infiltrator discovers that people feel the same tensions in most circumstances and institutional surroundings: am I alone or not alone? Am I OK or not? Does it all mean something or not? Am I loved or not?

Within a hospital the 'yes/no' waves are less easily suppressed than is possible elsewhere; it is this fact and this only which essentially distinguishes a hospital, and particularly a palliative care unit, from other human institutions. Suffering and the possibility of death bring a unique cutting edge to life's fundamental questions. There is no longer an escape from saying 'yes' to life or 'no' – even, and surely most importantly, to yourself.

A priest believes in saying 'yes' – not without confusion and recurring ambiguities – but 'yes'. Anywhere with people, he or she will try to help them discover life's 'yes' for themselves; he or she will be careful not to force choices or clutch at religious straws. Certainly God will not be offered 'neat'. The great hope is simply that a human being will say 'yes' in their own terms – God will be there too, on his – lovingly.

For an infiltrator in a palliative day care unit (and the chaplain who infiltrates may be a lay person rather than a priest) this seems to mean keeping a few essentials in the mind's eye. Oddly enough, they enter a chaplain's own spirituality and are brooded over in the inner quiet we call prayer.

The terms on which another lives

The 'yes' of a non-believer is as important as anyone else's; a thoughtful chaplain will rejoice in such a 'yes' in the midst of pain and fear and unbelief. Both chaplain and patient in such a relationship can advance towards their own particular 'yes' as they discuss and explore experience.

Similar sensitive partnerships can be entered by a Christian chaplain with members of other faiths as long as distinctive perspectives are known and respected; for example:

- Judaism is enormously life affirming, so for Jewish patients the use of the last days on this Earth is to be treasured and enjoyed.
- Hinduism nourishes acceptance, tolerance, a belief in rebirth and, ultimately, freedom through death.
- Islam means 'peaceful submission to God's will' and Allah is 'oft-forgiving and most merciful' in this relationship with the faithful Muslim.

The terms on which another works

With diffidence and respect a chaplain infiltrates the working lives of nurses and doctors and others who staff the palliative care unit. A chaplain does so with limited knowledge of the technicalities, but some awareness of the pain which is an inescapable part of competent caring . . . suffering shared with patients.

It is noticeable and surely right that a large proportion of a chaplain's time in a palliative care unit is simply offered in being with the staff.

The terms on which I infiltrate

When I arrive there is someone already there: we wait together until what is on their heart is spoken (if it ever is!):

I huddle warm inside my corner bed,
Watching the other patients sipping tea.
I wonder why I'm no longer getting well,
And why it is no one will talk to me.

The nurses are so kind. They brush my hair
On days I feel too ill to read or sew.
I smile and chat, try not to show my fear,
They cannot tell me what I want to know.

The visitors come in. I see their eyes
Become embarrassed as they pass my bed.
'What lovely flowers,' they say, then hurry on
In case their faces show what can't be said.

The chaplain passes on his weekly round
With friendly smile and calm, untroubled brow.
He speaks with sincerity of life,
I'd like to speak of death, but don't know how.

The surgeon comes in, with student retinue,
Mutters to Sister, deaf to my silent plea.
I want to tell this dread I feel inside,
But they are too kind to talk to me.

(Poem by a terminally ill patient, quoted by Olly McGilloway)[1]

In the end it is the 'yes' I listen for; the 'yes', for instance of a man in the unit I visit who on first seeing me, demonstrated that the way of survival involves ignoring the chaplain. After some weeks, we managed to nod to each other and eventually, finding ourselves sitting as neighbours in the centre, we became first, conversationalists and then, friends. Not many days before death, on his initiative the patient and his wife serenely received Holy Communion together; for him it was both the first and the last occasion.

It will not always be so; relationships are rarely tidy or the outcome of a chaplain's listening so obvious and moving. But it is the way chaplaincy is, and what is said of waiting with patients in this way is also true of waiting with their relatives.

The terms on which I understand myself

As the years pass I notice that the question of who is ministering to whom is less clear; regularly my tiredness is matched and soothed by a patient's concern for me. Again and again I witness lives fulfilled in chronic adversity, lives that previously seem to have been lacking in some quality or purpose. Any chaplain has repeatedly to face their own inner questionings and fears, their own feelings about dying and death. That this process is made more effective in a supervisory relationship, perhaps one with a spiritual director, is very apparent.

I am conscious also, that in the end, at the end, I will need others to minister to me, to assist me towards the possibility of saying my 'yes' in my terms.

Being practical

A chaplain is wise to be conscious of the wider world beyond the palliative day care centre, where the patient also lives a life; the greater part in fact. Linking a patient to others in that broader community is a significant contributor to appropriate spiritual care. Connecting or reconnecting a patient to a particular community of faith, if this is their wish, is a part of what may be appropriate.

Being chaplain is not a role which usually demands complex academic or technical competence; reflective and listening skills are the main tools of the trade. Books may be of particular help here.[2,3]

A final, recurring, question

A palliative care day centre unit is a strangely magnetic place; many of us are attracted to working in one and simply being there. This is good and natural, but it could easily become unbalanced. I have found, as a chaplain, that it is both necessary and probably healthy for me to keep asking myself this question: 'to what extent do I visit the terminally ill to reassure myself of my own strength and my own immortality, thereby denying my essential unity with those patients in their dying?'

References

1. McGilloway O. Nursing and spiritual care. In: Twycross RG, ed. *The dying patient*. CMF Publications, 1975.
2. McGilloway O, Myco F, eds. *Nursing and spiritual care*. London: Harper and Row, 1985.
3. Kubler-Ross E. *On death and dying*. London: Tavistock Publications, 1970.

Part V: Patient Services

17

Nutritional needs

Tim Hunt

Introduction

Food and drink are among the pleasures of life, and in some cases may become vices. Furthermore, they may assume greater importance when we are ill. However, illness brings about changes in many ways; the taste we associate with certain foods may change inexplicably; the smell of food being cooked is no longer an invitation to eat but may become repulsive; and what we previously could chew and swallow without effort may become difficult or impossible. Sometimes, the patient will describe these changing sensations, but frequently it may be someone else who first notices, as food is left on the plate and later when food is pushed away.

In illness there are three areas that influence our nutrition in practical terms:

1. The general symptoms associated with advanced cancer, as for example, the decrease in desire to eat and the gradual loss of weight.
2. Food preferences and the ability to eat may be determined by the type of cancer – obviously the effect of cancer of the stomach is different from that of an intracranial tumour.
3. The complex side-effects of treatment which may modify eating.

All these may affect our taste and preference, what we can and cannot eat and the value of food.

We will consider the more common changes experienced in illness that influence our eating and cause symptoms in advanced cancer; then we will consider some of the practical areas in looking after our patients.

The background

Anorexia

We do not understand fully why the desire to eat is often shut down in four out of five patients with cancer. This absence of the wish to eat is termed anorexia. There are complex and little-known biochemical changes in the body with most cancers and many tumours produce substances that promote anorexia. A number of chemical substances in the body are increased in cancer and these are known to diminish appetite. In addition there are other more easily understood changes that may contribute to anorexia – the dry mouth, the painful mouth and discomfort on swallowing; the frequent queasiness or nausea; depression and the diminishing social activity and enjoyment that are much a part of encouraging us to eat. Pharmacological substances are often used to stimulate appetite, the best known being the corticosteroids and progesterones, but often these drugs are short term in stimulating appetite and in the long term may cause many side-effects.

Weight loss

The loose dress hanging on the body and the collar that is far too large for the neck are frequent reminders that not all is well and provide a continual reminder of weight loss. The psychological consequences of this may cause considerable depression, because weight loss is visible evidence of fading life. There is no effective remedy to counteract this weight loss, although many ideas have been advanced and are used, including intensive feeding by mouth, intravenous lines and directly into the gastrointestinal tract. Total parenteral nutrition is to use these routes to provide liquid nutrients. Sadly none has a significant lasting effect on preventing a reduction in weight.

Nausea and vomiting

We are all too aware of vomiting because it is visible, but the sensation of nausea is a silent symptom and experienced by more than half the patients with cancer. The causes of nausea are legendary – they extend from anxiety and fear at the one extreme; through to liver involvement, decreased gastric and gut motility; they include infections and raised intracranial pressure as with tumours of the head; together with the side-effects of the very treatment we may use to alleviate symptoms. This may include drugs, radiotherapy and chemotherapy.

Despite the many causes of nausea, it is often impossible to establish the actual cause and it may require assiduous observation and detective work to establish possible associations; it may be the smell of certain food being cooked; the sight of the many medicines that have to be swallowed; travel in the car, and not least the anxiety from anticipating a medical investigation or even a consultation at which may be made known important results.

Nausea remains a major cause of preventing patients from eating and drinking those foods to which they are accustomed, and where the trigger is strong, as when certain foods are placed in front of the patient, the nausea gives way to a bout of uncontrolled vomiting. However, the fact that nausea and sometimes vomiting are associated with defined events, allows the careful observer the opportunity to take note and prevent their reoccurrence.

Change in taste

Patients are often aware of an alteration in their taste, but it may be someone else who notices that a previously favourite food is now discarded by the patient. These subtle changes in taste are complex and may be experienced in several ways. What was a pleasant taste previously may now be perceived as unpalatable, causing a symptom known as dysgeusia. In other cases, taste may become so diminished – hypogeusia – that all food tastes like cotton wool. In other circumstances, often associated with tumours of the brain, there may be episodes of having no taste – ageusia. In addition to these symptoms there may be frequent changes in what the patient may feel like eating, craving one day for a savoury food and the next day for a sweet food, as may be experienced in some pregnancies. This craving for some foods and distaste for others may reverse or change abruptly.

Some surgery or radiotherapy to the head and neck may have a temporary or permanent effect on taste. Likewise, bizarre changes in taste may be caused by therapy and drugs including the corticosteroids, hormonal preparations and chemotherapy. Although we do not know the mechanism that causes these changes, there are two important elements that are required to allow normal taste.

The taste buds. First, there must be adequate and active taste buds; these are found not only on the tongue, but are widely spread on the lips, the soft palate and other areas of the mouth and even extend to the upper oesophagus. In each of these areas the taste buds are tuned to help us to taste in a particular way. For example, the taste buds of the soft palate give us the main signals to discriminate sour and bitter tastes. However, this jigsaw that allows us our fine taste is further complicated by each taste bud having a regulator, which controls the sensitivity of the taste buds; this biochemical regulator, which allows molecules to be processed by the taste buds, is in turn affected by the changing biochemistry seen in patients with cancer. Therefore, not only may certain tastes be less sensitively perceived, (if one group of taste buds which specialises in a taste are out of full action), but the strength of taste may be diminished by abnormal biochemistry affecting the regulator of the taste buds.

Radiotherapy to the head and neck often causes a change in the perception of bitter and salt substances. These changes may return to near normal within 1 to 3 months, but may remain absent for 5 or more years before partial or full recovery. Some of the newer chemotherapeutic drugs may abruptly change taste sensation for a few days, while some of the commonly used hormonal preparations for prostatic cancer may considerably diminish the number of taste buds. While the loss or change in taste can follow numerous permutations, there are general trends such as salt in food tasting very much more salty.

The saliva. Second, the characteristics of saliva affect taste. Saliva is not an inert substance, but has a complex composition which is frequently changing according to our diet and illness which affect the salivary glands. Radiotherapy to the head and neck may result in more or less a complete loss of salivary production; many drugs may change the composition and flow of saliva, including corticosteroids, opioids, antiemetics and antidepressants.

The dry and sore mouth

The principal reason for problems in the mouth is because of changes in the composition and quantity of saliva. Saliva not only makes taste possible, as discussed above, but also lubricates the mouth and oropharynx. One important function of this is to allow food to be formed into a bolus so that the food can be swallowed, and the patient with a very dry mouth will often complain that the food 'sticks at the back of my throat'. There are more than sixty chemical substances in healthy saliva and some of these protect the mucosa of the mouth and gums from infection. The healthy salivary glands produce over a litre of rich salivary secretions each day. Usually these secretions are increased through a reflex as a result of the taste, sight, thought or smell of food. However, these stimuli are reduced in illness, so that there is a decreased secretion of saliva. There is a further decrease and change in saliva because many drugs and treatments reduce the function of the salivary glands.

The dry mouth is unprotected and vulnerable to trauma and infection; sometimes this is seen in the form of multiple or large single ulcers, which are further encouraged by the reduced immunological state of the body caused by disease or aggressive therapy.

The dry mouth feels heavy, swollen and uncomfortable which makes the entry of food and some drink both uncomfortable and tiresome. In extreme cases even speech becomes difficult, while with the loss of body weight there is atrophy of the gums that results in loose dentures, or the inability to wear dentures, which further adds to the many problems of the ill-functioning mouth.

Abdominal discomfort

The problems of eating and drinking are particularly encountered where a tumour, or secondary growth, involves the gastrointestinal tract. This may cause a multiplicity of symptoms where the wrong or excessive food is taken, but the effect of the tumour depends on where it is in the gut, and the pressure that it exerts on the hollow lumen, thereby causing a partial or complete mechanical blockage or obstruction.

Where the oesophagus is involved, the early problem is in swallowing bulky or dry foods. In many cases of oesophageal cancer, a rigid plastic tube may be inserted surgically to keep the oesophagus open. This allows a reasonable quantity of food and drink to be taken by mouth for some time. As the disease progresses, the surrounding tumour growth may occlude the lower end of the tube resulting in an obstruction, so that only some liquids may get through.

Some patients may experience a scalding or burning discomfort when they swallow liquids or food; this indicates possible inflammation of the oesophagus or upper stomach and may be so painful that attempts to eat or drink are stopped.

With gastric or stomach cancer, and growths near the outlet of the stomach, as seen in involvement of the pancreas or duodenum, the problem is that either the capacity of the stomach is diminished to accommodate food, or the rate at which food passes out of the stomach is slowed down. Subsequently, the patient will feel quickly bloated and often sick after taking a relatively small quantity of food or liquid. This may lead to explosive vomiting after which the patient feels more comfortable.

The liver is commonly involved from secondary spread in many cancers, and the changed biochemistry of the liver heightens the response to many stimuli, such as the sight or smell of food, which may cause nausea and vomiting.

Cancers involving the intestines, such as cancer of the colon, may slowly occlude the lumen of the gut and cause simple mechanical obstruction. The macerated food and liquid is unable to pass this obstruction and may build up above this point to cause nausea and often considerable pain. The patient may feel so unwell that drinking and eating are not even considered. These mechanical problems may be made worse by the type of food, and as the tumour prevents the normal propulsion of food along the gut, there is abnormal stretching of the gut which may cause pain. Air that we swallow when talking and eating may become entrapped in parts of the gut, causing more pain.

Constipation

In many cases of cancer one of the commonest symptoms is that of constipation. This is found frequently where a person is receiving medication, such as analgesics to reduce pain, and nearly all analgesics may cause constipation. The constipated person may feel uncomfortable and unwell in several ways, including a feeling of nausea, abdominal distension and pain, and even confusion has been known in the elderly. Considering correct nutrition is important in preventing constipation.

Practical considerations

Explanation and education

Patients know when they feel sick or when they have problems in swallowing, but seldom do they have any idea about what is causing these problems. Thoughtful and sympathetic explanation may help, especially where the patient and relatives may be responsible for food and drink, and it is important to discuss the problems with them, especially where a change in their eating may reduce their symptoms.

The mouth

The mouth needs both lubrication and stimulation; lubrication to protect the mouth and stimulation to encourage the reflexes that activate the salivary glands to produce more saliva.

Lubrication. Lubrication of the mouth is made possible by the saliva, which keeps it moist and healthy. When the supply of saliva is poor, it may help to use proprietary artificial saliva. However, these are poor substitutes for natural, healthy saliva. An economical and useful mucilage is a methylcellulose in water solution (10 g in 1 litre) which can be enhanced by the addition of a small amount of citric acid. The citric acid acts as a salivary stimulant. Previously many of the larger hospitals had their own formulation for making such preparations which were given the name of the hospital, as for example the Westminster Solution. The mucilage is best kept in a refrigerator. Because it clings to the mucosa of the mouth, it has an advantage over sips of water. Carmellose can also be used as the main base. Mucilages can be prepared by a helpful local pharmacist. Another useful idea is the sucking of soft gum pastilles that do not contain medication.

Stimulating saliva. The function of the salivary glands is often depressed because of medication, and for this reason it is important to regularly review medication where the patient complains of a dry mouth.

Saliva may be stimulated by the use of aperitifs taken 30 minutes before a meal. The best examples of these are the dry versions of Vermouth, Pastis and Dubonnet. These also stimulate the gastric juices which may help some patients. A chilled, dry white wine or chilled, unsweetened dry sherry, are good substitutes. Other stimulatory foods include clear bouillon, from which the fat has been skimmed off, and which is taken about 30 minutes before the meal. Likewise, drinks containing aromatic bitters, such as tonic water which contains quinine, are stimulants. The simple action of chewing an apple, which may be easier to eat if cut into slices, causes a four-fold increase in saliva for a short time.

Mouth ulcers. Where there are mouth ulcers the mucosa needs protection; otherwise acidic drinks or foods, such as citric juices or tomatoes, cause a burning or smarting around the ulcer. Large, painful ulcers may make moving the mouth uncomfortable when chewing or talking. The ulcer should be covered with a light film of petroleum jelly ('Vaseline') which may be used several times a day and applied especially before taking food or drink. Seldom is there a need to use special medicaments; petroleum jelly works well, is almost tasteless, and is not washed away by water or alcohol.

Mouth washes. There are a number of proprietary mouth washes and preparations containing anaesthetic agents to ameliorate the painful mouth, and these may have a role. However, many are acidic and may further hurt and delay healing of the ulcerated mouth. The fundamental approach is to keep the mouth clean, moist and protected and not camouflage the source of discomfort by using a topical anaesthetic agent. A weak solution of hydrogen peroxide mouth wash provides an uplifting and fresh feeling, and is an excellent cleansing agent, but ulcers should first be protected before using this. Pineapple is advocated for the mouth because of an enzyme contained in this fruit, but the acidic nature may aggravate the traumatised mouth. Less acidic is the papaya (paw-paw) fruit which contains a similar enzyme.

Painful and difficult swallowing

Discomfort or pain on swallowing food or drink often indicates an inflammatory state of the oesophagus, and a soothing demulcent often helps. Demulcents include methylcellulose mucilage; milk with a high fat content; the white of a raw egg mixed with milk; lignocaine and hydrocortisone mouth wash which may be swallowed in small quantities; and, an antacid containing a local anaesthetic such as oxethazine. These should be swallowed slowly 10–20 minutes before taking solids or drinks. They are especially useful following radiotherapy to the chest or thorax which may cause transient inflammation of the oesophagus.

In cancers of the oesophagus or stomach, the general rule is to prepare food in a wet or liquid state, according to individual tolerance, and to take small quantities of food and drink at a time. When food is wet, or in a liquid form, it is easier for it to get past a stricture than it would be for dry or bulky food such as a roast potato. However, some fluids, such as water, are not easily carried down a dysfunctioning oesophagus, and in these cases a heavier liquid, such as milk, is managed more easily. Where solid food can no longer be taken, food can be provided in a jus de viande or smooth sauce. The function of a sauce, whether from meat or vegetables, is to provide a food that is both nutritious and which may be swallowed easily. A warm, brown or white sauce is most effective because a warm sauce is an excellent lubricant. Even a sauce that is part of a dish itself, as with coq au vin or chicken chasseur, is both nutritious and tolerated more easily.

Other alternatives that provide high nutritional intake and lubrication are home-made stock, or proprietary stock cubes diluted to taste. If the stricture is advanced, a fine liquidiser should be used to prepare the food.

Where an oesophageal tube has been inserted, it is usual for the hospital to give patients a leaflet explaining suitable foods. The aim is to avoid food that may stick and obstruct the tube as this will mean admission to hospital to unblock it. These instructions should be followed before preparing food for the patient. Aerated waters, such as soda water, are often used after each meal to keep the tube free of debris and to unblock it.

Discomfort after eating and drinking

A tumour or stricture in the oesophagus, stomach or intestine often means that the ability to deal with normal quantities of food and drink is considerably reduced. This may be indicated by either a delay in the usual time it takes to swallow, and from remarks such as 'it won't go down', or a feeling of upper abdominal fullness, sometimes with pain, very soon after eating a small quantity of food. While wet and liquid foods are tolerated more easily, the rule is to offer smaller portions of food and drink. This should be explained to the patient, using perhaps reference to a partly blocked plumbing system, along which it takes longer for liquids to pass through. With this information, the patient may understand better the reason for adjusting their eating habits.

A full or bloated feeling is often experienced in cases of gut cancer, and some general guidelines should be considered. Drinks containing gas should be drunk in moderation, and the gas can be reduced by using a swirl-stick to disperse it. A careful watch should be kept on which foods may bring about discomfort. Many vegetables and fruits are frequently implicated, including members of the cabbage family, beans, and to a lesser extent apples, grapes, raisins and even bananas. Orange is seldom implicated, but fruits such as oranges and tangerines, which may have strong segments, must be chewed or the segment split open so that the segment is not swallowed whole. A large segment is seldom broken down once it is swallowed and may block a stricture of the gut.

Taste, smell and sight of food

Taste preferences for a patient should be established at frequent intervals, as these may change every few days. It is difficult to generalise about taste preferences, as the liking for some tastes is a very individual matter.

The smell of food may often trigger a bout of nausea; this is especially associated with the volatile smells given off when cooking meat, particularly from frying. Every effort should be made to prevent cooking smells from wafting to the patient. Even when warm food is on the plate, the smell from some meats and vegetables (for example Brussels sprouts give off sulphur when cooked), may induce nausea and subsequent vomiting. If patients are very sensitive to such smells, it is better to consider serving cold meat and vegetables.

The flavour of most foods comes essentially from the fat content, and many who are ill find it repulsive. Seasoned meat eaters want to continue eating meat which they regard as an essential for life, but often it is the cooking and eating of meat that promotes nausea. The lean and white meats, with up to about 10 per cent fat, such as chicken, are best tolerated when ill; while the semi-lean meats, with up to 20 per cent fat, as in certain cuts of beef, lamb and turkey, are less well tolerated. The fatty meats with more than 20 per cent fat, such as pork and some cuts of beef and lamb, may need to be avoided where there is the slightest suspicion of nausea. However, it is not only the type of meat that dictates the fat content but the method of cooking. Therefore, by careful and appropriate cooking, and by draining off the fat that has collected during cooking, meat previously considered fatty may be acceptable. Boiling and stewing increase the tenderness of meat.

The sight of food may cause a patient to feel more unwell because of a past association with that food, from an occasion when tasting it caused them to feel unwell. It may be difficult to break this association, and if there is no explanation for this, then that food must be gently reintroduced in small amounts. Some food substances change their biochemical structure when warmed or cooked and are less tolerated than if served cold; milk is a good example of a substance that shows these changes. The sight of a plate piled high is unappetising to most patients; it is better to serve small quantities and offer further servings. The smell of food is less noticeable from smaller portions. Colour of food may also deter a patient from wanting to eat; certain yellow and brown coloured foods may trigger early stages of nausea, but it may be that it is not any individual colour, but more a large expanse of colour on the plate that is viewed as unaesthetic and unappetising by the patient.

Where nausea and vomiting have taken place recently it may help to offer dry biscuits, such as cream crackers, or even soft toast, as such dry substances seem to placate the tendency to further nausea and vomiting.

Alcohol

The labelling on medicine reads frequently that alcohol should not be taken together with that medicine; there are sensible reasons for this as some drugs interact with alcohol to make a person feel sleepy and this may cause problems in driving or operating machinery. Nevertheless, alcohol is an important beverage and an opportunity for social interchange for many people. As such it is churlish to deny it to patients who have for many years regarded it as part of their normal life. Throughout the centuries alcohol has been given in various forms for therapeutic purposes and while this will be the subject of debate for many more centuries, it gives pleasure to many and should be offered with this in mind.

Fluids and hydration

Insufficient emphasis is given to providing and encouraging the drinking of more fluid. We need about 2 litres of fluid a day, three quarters of that being obtained from drinking fluid and one quarter from the water contained in the food we eat. Most people drink and eat far less when they are ill. Inadequate fluid intake is the commonest contributing cause of constipation, which is itself a major problem in our patients. A further need for more fluid is seen in the many patients who experience bouts of sweating, because of their illness, and this fluid loss needs to be replaced by additional fluid intake. It is imperative to give far greater emphasis to increasing the intake of fluid and to encourage this; each element needs to be made more attractive – from the taste and temperature of the water, to considering additions to the water to vary the taste, and not forgetting the water container and the drinking glass.

Supplements

A plethora of nutritional supplements is available and these are given frequently to patients. We do not know what is the ideal nutritional supplement for the patient with cancer, but current thinking suggests that there should be a reasonably high intake of protein. Protein-rich foods are not only found in meat products but also as vegetable proteins, such as vegetable stocks. Dairy products are rich in protein, contain sufficient fat to provide an attractive taste, and allow the food to be prepared and served in many ways. The continual taking of the more frequently prescribed nutritional supplements soon becomes boring and unpleasant, and probably more attractive tastes and textures can be obtained from individual home-prepared recipes. Vitamin supplements may be encouraged, particularly vitamin C (ascorbic acid), but again we are uncertain about the full benefits of these supplements. There is a new interest in the suggested benefit of fish oil preparations, and continual interest in the value of mineral supplements. Our overall state of knowledge suggests that we should supplement food where the food intake provides less than 1500 kilocalories a day.

Conclusions

There are many dilemmas and unknown factors about food and feeding for the patient who is ill with cancer. We know that much of the food that is eaten is not synthesised as in the healthy person, leading to low levels of protein in the muscles and alteration in the normal breakdown and use of carbohydrates, but we do not understand the many and complex reasons that may bring about these changes. Despite the provision of considerable supplementary nutrition in different ways, it remains difficult to correct this disturbed synthesis of food; weight will continue to be lost and weakness supervenes. For the majority, the meaning of food as an essential for the continuation of life must remain and the thoughts of patients and relatives should be addressed. It may mean sensitive discussion to explain to a patient that some adjustment is required in their eating habits. It is important to provide food and drink that can be accepted and tolerated by our patients, that may even in a small way enhance their feeling of well-being and ameliorate where possible some of their symptoms. Above all, food and drink should give pleasure. The technology of food and nutrition must take second place and the personal likes and dislikes should take first place. That is the key in caring for all patients.

18

Physiotherapy

Lydia Gillham

Has physiotherapy a role in palliative care?

The fact is that physiotherapists have worked in day care centres for almost as long as the profession has been in existence. However, the involvement of the physiotherapist working in a palliative day care centre is still a relatively new development. It is useful therefore to take some time to consider the best possible ways in which physiotherapists can contribute. In order to do this a clear understanding of their role is essential.

The impact of variations in working practice

There is a widespread agreement in palliative care units that the patient benefits most when a well coordinated 'team' delivers the care. Physiotherapists in common with other professionals may be affiliated to several different teams at the same time. However, being human they are likely to identify most with the team which provides their 'home base'. This may be where they are employed or 'where they hang up their coat'. This simple allegiance in the mind will have important effects on the physiotherapist in terms of time, access to equipment and professional accountability.

Considerable variations exist in the employment situation of physiotherapists. They may undertake their day care work:

- exclusively for the day care unit;
- in combination with other duties relating to out-patients and in-patients within a hospice;
- as a modest part of their total case load as a physiotherapist in a general hospital;
- as a community physiotherapist dealing with individual patients either when they are attending the day care centre, or when they are in their own home;
- as a specialist palliative community physiotherapist, where the day care centre is part of a more extensive work load.

Skilled physiotherapy is a rare commodity and most of the situations described above are unlikely to provide much time for 'hands on' treatment. Time management practices need to be employed and skills relating to treatment and management passed on to other people wherever feasible. The day-to-day practice of a programme of exercises can often be absorbed into a daily routine and supervised if necessary by someone other than the physiotherapist.

Can conventional physiotherapy cope with palliative day care?

In some respects working in palliative care resembles working in other areas such as neurology, orthopaedics and surgery. Indeed many of the patients eventually referred to the day centre will have attended such units first and the knowledge and skills developed there are certainly relevant to the work of palliative day care units.

The basic skills of a physiotherapist which are easily transferred from other contexts to the day care situation include:

- extracting relevant information from records and other people to use as a 'background' prior to seeing a patient;
- assessing the overall situation and selecting appropriate examination procedures;
- assessing and carrying out an examination of the patient;
- devising an appropriate physiotherapy programme;
- teaching appropriate basic physiotherapy skills to carers and monitoring them;
- selecting and applying treatments which require specific physiotherapy training;
- evaluating and continually adjusting the programme.

Despite this impressive range of transferable skills, physiotherapists who choose to specialise in palliative care will find it essential to gather new knowledge and develop additional skills in certain areas. For example new areas of expertise in oncology, methods of palliation and the processes of grief and loss will have to be developed.[1]

What are the key differences for the physiotherapist in palliative care?

There seem to be four key areas of difference for the physiotherapist considering a move into palliative care. These are changes in thinking to be accomplished; the acceptance of a different professional image; the need to cope with a complex admixture of pleasure and pain inherent in the work; and the need to develop a professional approach to patients which may, on occasions, resemble that of a counsellor.

Developing a different way of thinking

In so many areas of clinical practice health professionals are persuasively inducted into thinking curatively. Most physiotherapists have come to feel more comfortable with this; for example, physiotherapists working in areas such as sports injuries deal with patients who are able to cooperate with very active and demanding exercises in the secure knowledge that, before too long, they will return to normal function again. Moving from areas like this into palliative care requires a shift in perception and a different way of thinking. There is a need to develop a positive approach to situations which can often appear extremely bleak.[2]

In addition, the palliative care physiotherapist is soon made aware that the view of their job seen from the outside is very different from reality. To the outsider, palliative care may appear to be about 'working with dying patients'. In practice, it is about working with living patients and improving their quality of life whenever possible. The palliative care physiotherapist will be engaged for most of the time in active and practical work in the pursuit of the best possible quality of life for patients whose remaining time is likely to be limited.

Fostering a different image

All health professionals have to live with the image that other people have of them and of their profession. Sometimes that image can be helpful and at other times a hindrance which the professional must come to terms with. A common perception of the physiotherapist is of someone who 'pushes' people into doing things that they don't want to do – 'a physioterrorist', as someone once described it! This view of the physiotherapist may prevent people wanting to undertake a programme of physiotherapy, or cooperating with it. To be effective the physiotherapist needs to be ready to recognise and accept that individual patients may perceive them in a negative way. It then becomes possible to work towards creating a different image in which the physiotherapist is seen as someone who, whilst being kind, gentle, and making perfectly reasonable demands, achieves highly beneficial results.

Coping with the pain and the pleasure

The palliative care physiotherapist works with a case load of patients whose abilities are likely to decline over the period of their contact. Whilst progressive deterioration can be a feature in many areas of physiotherapy work, in palliative care it is presented more starkly. Not only will the decline be faster but it is likely to end in the death of more patients. This realistic background is compounded by the fact that patients frequently have expectations about what physiotherapy can do for them which are highly unrealistic and uncomfortable. The patient's unwritten agenda that 'this physiotherapist will get me walking again' can be a considerable source of stress for the professional. In order to survive it without emotional burnout, the physiotherapist must be honest and at the same time aware of their own human reactions and those that the patient is displaying. Acting otherwise is likely to generate even higher levels of stress. All these painful needs must be balanced against the job satisfaction experienced when physiotherapy intervention leads to improvements in patient morale and functional abilities and makes a real contribution to the 'end quality' of a declining life.

Moving towards a counselling approach

In a day care setting physiotherapists spend a considerable time relating face-to-face with individual patients. Because of this, and the intimacy it engenders, they are often drawn into situations which involve handling very difficult questions:

'Will I get the use of my legs back?'
'How long do you think I'll be able to go on doing this?'

Early professional training in physiotherapy rarely provides adequate preparation for responding to questions like these. Because of this, physiotherapists in this kind of work often choose to extend their training into counselling skills.[3] Such training helps to improve their capacity for listening, attending and reflecting. However, physiotherapists need to bear in mind that they are not counsellors *per se*. Physiotherapists are not counsellors with a big 'C', and are more likely to use a modest small 'c' counselling approach in their personal interactions with each patient.

Realistic contributions from the physiotherapist

Most physiotherapists entering the field of palliative care need more than a simple specification of how they need to change. Above all, they need to be convinced that they are going to make a unique and valuable contribution to the care team. This notion of making an effective contribution is at the heart of team-based palliative care. Accordingly, here are some of the important contributions which the physiotherapist can make.

Contribution 1: planning realistic programmes for patients

Patients attending a day care unit will often be referred to the physiotherapist in order to assist in the planning of a 'rehabilitation programme'.

Rehabilitation involves a team effort and depends upon the contribution made by all the professionals involved. There are few people working in palliative care who do not recognise the importance of rehabilitation and the power exerted by the word itself. All patients should be given the opportunity of rehabilitation. Dietz in his book *Rehabilitation oncology*[4] strongly recommends the use of this word in the treatment of cancer patients because it fosters a positive and hopeful approach to programme planning. He proposes that for the wider spectrum of disabilities the goals set for patients should fall into four different rehabilitation categories:

- preventative
- restorative
- supportive
- palliative.

These four categories have provided a satisfactory way of thinking for most professionals working in palliative care. However, the negative side of the coin is that many professionals faced by a patient who is obviously deteriorating find that the word rehabilitation does not fit comfortably with reality, even when their goals are palliative ones. This is because the word itself often conjures up restoration in the minds of patients and can lead to unrealistic expectations which are doomed to disappointment.

This has led the author of this chapter to adopt the alternative term 'active readaptation'.[5] It seems that Dietz's rejection of 're-adaptation' and the decision to sink it in the notion of rehabilitation was psychologically and linguistically flawed. It was flawed because the unrealistic connotations put on the word 'rehabilitation', by some patients and palliative care professionals, can be overpowering. By contrast, the term proposed here seeks to combine the realism of re-adaptation with the optimism of the word 'active'. Here, the emphasis is on an active response, even though the essential problem is acknowledged. This phrase, which does not imply a passive acceptance of the situation, is likely to be more meaningful for some physiotherapists working with palliative care patients. Active re-adaptation implies that the patient is encouraged to continually adapt to new circumstances as they gradually lose abilities and functions. Unlike Dietz, I do not believe 're-adaptation' is simply a synonym for 'rehabilitation'.

All that I have said so far about planning – particularly for patients who are very ill – will help to ensure that treatment programmes are carefully and appropriately constructed without being unrealistic. In effect, I am saying that approaching the situation from the standpoint of active re-adaptation will help all members of the care team to go through a stage of systematically 'thinking through the situation' as it is, rather than as they wish it to be.

Yoshioka carried out a study of the rehabilitation of more than 300 patients with advanced cancer over a period of six and a half years. He showed that rehabilitation is capable of making an important contribution to the care and well-being of patients with very advanced cancer. One of his most useful findings was that the more fully patients were involved in discussing their physical programme with the therapist the more effective and satisfactory the rehabilitation proved to be.[6]

These activities of 'thinking it through' and 'negotiating the programme' are illustrated in Figure 18.1.

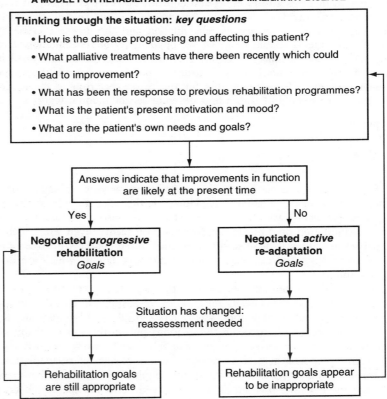

A MODEL FOR REHABILITATION IN ADVANCED MALIGNANT DISEASE

Thinking through the situation: *key questions*

- How is the disease progressing and affecting this patient?
- What palliative treatments have there been recently which could lead to improvement?
- What has been the response to previous rehabilitation programmes?
- What is the patient's present motivation and mood?
- What are the patient's own needs and goals?

Answers indicate that improvements in function are likely at the present time

Yes

No

Negotiated *progressive* **rehabilitation**
Goals

Negotiated *active* **re-adaptation**
Goals

Situation has changed: reassessment needed

Rehabilitation goals are still appropriate

Rehabilitation goals appear to be inappropriate

Fig. 18.1 Rehabilitation and active re-adaptation.

Another difficulty in rehabilitation is in choosing a satisfactory measurement tool, which can demonstrate the effectiveness of the outcome of a treatment programme.[7] Because rehabilitation can cover so many different aspects of the patient's life and involves so many professionals, it isn't surprising that there are estimated to be over 10 000 tests available for use. However, there are several key principles which are of over-arching importance, whatever specific instruments are selected for assessing these patients. There is a need:

- to concentuate on quality of life
- to be sensitive and non-invasive
- to use instruments which are both valid and reliable.

Contribution 2: providing equipment which is sensitively related to patient need

Providing equipment which has been properly assessed for a specific patient can have a liberating effect. It can help the patient to achieve independence in functional activities such as walking, eating and reading. Conversely, if such equipment is provided at the wrong time to the wrong patient, it can have highly negative effects. In circumstances where the professional feels helpless, there is a temptation to deal with these feelings by giving equipment to the patient. As a result, patients may be provided with too many pieces of equipment. The problem is compounded when the equipment is not removed when it is no longer used. The result can be too much clutter, which can obscure the patient's real needs. In the advanced stages of diseases such as cancer, each new aid confronts the patient with the inescapable fact that they have deteriorated further, and because of this, equipment – new or otherwise – needs to be provided sensitively, following a careful assessment.

Wheelchairs, in particular, need to be provided in a sensitive way. Patients often see their move into a wheelchair as a 'stage' to be avoided. As a consequence of this natural reluctance, their mobility will be increasingly restricted by the distance they can walk, and their world similarly limited. The option of leaving the provision of a wheelchair until the last possible moment has certain other disadvantages. By this time, the patient will be even more ill than before, and less likely to cope with learning a new skill. For patients, the point at which they cease to be ambulant and become wheelchair mobile can seem sudden and clearly demarcated. This can often be avoided by providing wheelchairs much earlier, for patients to explore whilst they are still ambulant. The transition between ambulant and wheelchair mobility then becomes less clear-cut. It is also important

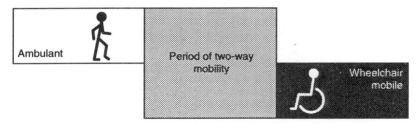

Fig. 18.2 Introducing wheelchairs – blurring the transition.

to watch the language used. Thinking in terms of patients being wheelchair mobile rather than wheelchair bound can be very useful.

One successful approach to introducing wheelchairs to patients is to emphasise that they must continue to exercise and walk around, but to encourage them to consider using a wheelchair for longer distances. This reassures them that accepting the wheelchair won't make them lose the ability to walk, and that the wheelchair can help them to conserve their energy.

Contribution 3: giving advice on mobility, and exercise

Mobility in some shape or form is necessary to preserve the quality of life. To enjoy doing things, patients need to be able to move around. Day centres often plan their days around activities, either within the centre or by providing trips outside. Whilst physiotherapy sessions involving contrived exercises have their value, purposeful exercise which is 'inbuilt' into social activities within and outside the centre is likely to be much more successful.

The physiotherapist is very frequently the person asked to advise on how much exercise is appropriate. Patients are anxious, both about doing too much and about doing too little. Because of this, the palliative care physiotherapist needs to be aware of several factors which may reduce the patient's ability to undertake exercises.

It is not surprising that patients are unmotivated towards exercise, particularly when their sleep has been disturbed by pain, symptoms or anxiety. The words, 'I can't be bothered to do anything' can also be related to general weakness and tiredness, resulting from poor nutrition which may in turn be related to nausea, vomiting or the invasion of the gastro–intestinal tract by disease.

Patients often complain that, '... my legs feel weak'. Such muscle weakness may simply be due to lack of exercise. But understandably, if patients have been feeling unwell for some time, they may have avoided activity or even been encouraged to 'sit down and rest'.

Of course, in advanced cancer, a number of other explanations are possible. For example, some drugs may have caused proximal weakness, or alternatively, nerves may be compressed by a tumour. Also, when distal groups are involved, there is always the danger of a cord compression. The physiotherapist is well placed to detect early signs of this serious 'emergency' complication. Muscle weakness may also result from the failure or reduced efficiency of major organs such as the heart, kidneys and liver. Other systemic causes include urinary and chest infections, or paraneoplastic syndrome.

Contribution 4: helping with the lifting, handling, moving and positioning of patients

The main import of the literature and legislation about lifting patients is to avoid doing it whenever possible! The physiotherapist is likely to be the person who is allocated the task of facilitating safe handling procedures in palliative care units. This involves making an initial assessment of the risks posed by the movement of a particular patient. Current legislation requires that the risk and the recommended lifting methods used are recorded so that everyone can follow good practice. The palliative care team requires a practical document which is comprehensive, and yet not *so* detailed as to be unworkable (a sample document is presented in Appendix 1). Day care necessarily involves a lot of movement of patients – for example, into and out of wheelchairs, easy chairs, toilets, and cars. To make this manageable, a variety of good equipment and regular teaching sessions on practical skills are essential.

All physiotherapists are trained in methods of lifting, handling and moving patients, and in the assessment of the risks involved for carers. However, the patients in palliative care have particular problems which need special consideration, too. For example, the presence of bone cancer and associated pain relief carries the risk of pathological fractures. Indeed, the presence of fractures can also make safe transfers difficult. In addition, tumours, skin cancers, wounds and tenderness to touch can sometimes make traditional methods of movement and methods of holding patients difficult to apply. In concentrating on movement, the therapist should not lose sight of the fact that good positioning can also ease and prevent pain.[8]

Contribution 5: offering advice on complementary and comfort therapies

Many health professionals in palliative care including physiotherapists are interested in the contributions which complementary therapy can make to the well-being of their patients. Most of these people are particularly interested in 'comfort therapies', which frequently involve touching the patient and clearly generate a 'feel good' factor.[9] However, incautious claims about 'curing' and 'healing' should be treated with circumspection. The need for these complementary therapy skills and the number of people willing to train and practise them is certainly increasing rapidly, and there is little doubt that they do make a real contribution to the patient's quality of life. This burgeoning of provision makes it vitally important that palliative care units develop policies which protect patients from excessive claims, and yet provide the opportunity of access to complementary therapies. Such policies should provide for screening of the qualifications, expertise and motivations of the therapists. In some centres, the introduction of a Complementary Therapy Panel has proved a useful initiative. This sort of panel could oversee development, monitor the type of therapies available and assess the personnel involved in this expanding area, offering advice and guidance when appropriate (a document detailing some early thinking about the place of complementary therapies in palliative care is included in Appendix 2).

Contribution 6: providing consultancy and education beyond the palliative care unit

The physiotherapist in the day care unit will in time develop special expertise in palliative care, and will begin to operate as a resource for those outside. Advice on palliative care issues in general and on specific matters relating to individual patients becomes an important part of the daily workload. This educational dimension should not be neglected if the principles practised within the unit are to be taken outside to inform practice within the broader health care community. Because of the expansion and changing nature of palliative care, it is in the interests of all those concerned to foster an environment which encourages other professionals to drop in for advice and support.

The necessary facilities for palliative physiotherapy

The physiotherapy service will be greatly enhanced by the provision of high-quality, specialist facilities and appropriate equipment.[10]

The treatment room is likely to be the hub of the enterprise. This room should have an 'open door' policy, and be accessible independently, to ambulant patients and those in wheelchairs. In these circumstances, patients can be encouraged to make use of the facilities several times a day, and undertake exercise sessions. Exercise 'a little at a time and often' is particularly appropriate for patients suffering from advanced disease, who are likely to tire easily. The space provided should be sufficient to make it possible for several patients to be actively involved at one time. Physiotherapy treatment might then become a 'social event', enhanced by positive features such as sharing, caring, commiserating, and encouraging.

Providing occupational therapy and physiotherapy in one treatment room would help to coordinate these two services. Calling the room the 'Rehabilitation and Therapy Room' would further enhance the provision by conjuring an active image combined with a sense of direction. Names are important, because they have the power to alter the perceptions of patients and professionals alike – words can radically affect the way people think, communicate and act.

Access to hydrotherapy facilities can add a further dimension to rehabilitation services. For some patients, being in water is a pleasure, but sensitivity is essential, as for some patients, immersion in water is certainly not pleasurable! Nevertheless, for most patients, the warmth and comfort provided by the water can be useful for relaxation. Water can be used both as a way of making exercise easier by reducing weight and assisting movement, and, conversely, as a way of making things more difficult by creating mild resistance. Hydrotherapy can also provide a useful medium for the performance of passive exercises, for gaining confidence in standing and providing practice in walking. In these circumstances, handling is made easier for the physiotherapist because the water provides a lot of support. The buoyancy of the water also provides weight relief, thereby relieving pains which are due to weight bearing.[11]

Conclusion

From the foregoing, it is readily apparent that the physiotherapist can make a useful contribution to the management of patients in the palliative day care unit. The physiotherapist is employed to best effect when other team members understand and appreciate the way in which they work, their values, their logical approach to treatment, and the feelings they have about their role in palliative care.

For the future, there is a need for basic education in palliative care to be introduced into undergraduate physiotherapy courses in higher education. There should also be enhanced opportunities for further development at postgraduate level to provide research skills. A number of areas of research seem particularly important. Firstly, there is a need to investigate patterns of exercise and mobility for patients with advanced malignant disease, and current models of rehabilitative and re-adaptative palliative care need to be evaluated more systematically.

References

1. Association of Chartered Physiotherapists in Oncology and Palliative Care. *Physiotherapy in oncology and palliative care – guidelines for good practice* (1993), available from The Chartered Society of Physiotherapy, 14 Bedford Row, London, WC1R 4ED.
2. Gray RC. Physiotherapy. In: Doyle D, Hanks GWC, McDonald N, eds *Oxford textbook of palliative medicine*. Oxford: Oxford University Press, 1993; 530–5.
3. Saunders C, Maxwell M. The case for counselling in physiotherapy: *Physiotherapy* 1987; **17**(11): 592–5.
4. Dietz JH, ed. *Rehabilitation oncology*. New York: John Wiley, 1981.
5. Gillham L. Palliative care: In: Pickles B, ed. *Physiotherapy with older people*. London: WB Saunders, 1995; 305–22.
6. Yoshioka H. Rehabilitation for the terminal cancer patient: *Amer J Phys Med Rehab* 1994; **73**(3).
7. Fulton CL. Measures of rehabilitation status in oncology: *Physiotherapy* 1994; **8**(12): 849–53.
8. Regnard C, Thompson J. *Controlling the pain*. A St Oswald's Open Learning Guide: Unit I, 1994; 23–31.
9. Sims S. The significance of touch in palliative care: *Palliative Med* 1988; **2**: 58–61.
10. Gillham L. *Improving the physiotherapy service: a fact sheet from the Hospice Infomation Service*, St Christopher's Hospice, London, 1994.
11. Skinner AT, Thompson AM. Hydrotherapy in pain: In: Wells PE, Frampton V, Bowsher D, eds. *Pain: Management by physiotherapy*, 2nd edn. Oxford: Butterworth–Heinemann, 1994; 228–37.

Appendix 1: Assessment and guidance on lifting and handling

Name of patient   *Date*   *Initials*

A This patient has been assessed and does not need
   help from staff at the present time. *If this is your*
   decision, you need go no further on this form. However,
   you may need to review the situation periodically.

B To be completed by any competent profession for
   patients requiring *manual* or *mechanical* help from staff
   with movement.

Assessment of risk to staff   *Date*   *Initials*

Weight: exact if known   Tick
                     estimate if not known   as appropriate
   below 5 stone   ❏
   5–8 stone   ❏
   8–12 stone   ❏
   12–16 stone   ❏
   16–25 stone   ❏
   25 stone and over   ❏

NB: special hoists need to be hired for patients
weighing 25 stone or more.

Reasons why patients may constitute a risk to staff during lifting and handling

The patient: Tick
• physically has difficulty or is unable   if appropriate
  to assist due to
  ....   ❏

• psychologically has difficulties or is
  unable to assist because   ❏

• has insufficient or no sitting balance
  ....   ❏

• has insufficient or no energy to assist
  due to ....   ❏

• normal holds are difficult or not
  possible because
  ....   ❏

• other ....   ❏

Advice and guidance

Use the following equipment

Tick
if appropriate

- Sara hoist   ❑
- Maxilift – small/medium/large sling   ❑
- Transfer board   ❑
  banana/straight/lateral
- Turntable   ❑
- Easyglide   ❑
- Medisling   ❑
- Transfer belt   ❑
- Lifting belt or harness   ❑
- Drawsheet/lifting net   ❑
- Monkey pole   ❑
- Other   ❑

....
....

- None of these   ❑

Use the following techniques

- No manual lift alone is appropriate   ❑
- Australian lift   ❑
- Through arm lift   ❑
- Standing transfer   ❑
- Sitting transfer   ❑
- Draw sheet lift   ❑
- Other   ❑

....
....

Other advice likely to be helpful

....
....
....
....

Appendix 2: Early work in establishing a complementary therapy policy

Stages recommended

It was suggested that there were probably three stages necessary to establish and implement a satisfactory policy.

1. To establish a resource file

This should be readily available for reference and will include:

- Agreed policy and guidelines.
- Useful addresses, e.g. British Complementary Association.
- Details of courses in complementary therapy to include training details and qualifications where appropriate. These could be used for reference when a practitioner applies to work in the hospice, either as a volunteer or staff.
- Names and telephone numbers of practitioners representing different therapies who have agreed to be approached for advice.
- Bibliographies and useful references.

2. To make recommendations to management

- A 'complementary therapy panel' of three people should be established. It should if possible include representations from the voluntary, clinical and complementary therapy areas. The panel could:
  - Maintain an up-to-date list of therapies and therapists, staff and volunteers already operating in the hospice. This would control the number of practitioners using a particular therapy.
  - Recommend which therapists could be introduced initially and help to rationalise the overall use.
  - Design an application form for therapists.
- A policy document be prepared which would outline a procedure for applicants and guidelines for working in the hospice.
- That this document should be put out for consultation.
- That this document should be put into a standard policy format.

3. To establish a policy for the practice of complementary therapy

The outline features of viable policy would include:

Applicants will be required to complete an application form containing details of:

- Courses they have attended, details of content, qualifications gained, updating.
- Their experience of using their particular therapy, in particular any clinical areas of work which are similar to the hospice.
- The potential benefits, contra-indications and precautions for their therapy.
- The objectives they are pursuing in using their therapy with the patients in the hospice.
- How they intend to work e.g. one-off sessions, courses of treatment, etc.

Applicants will attend an interview and:

- Bring certificates of qualifications.
- Bring a certificate of insurance cover.
- Supply references – character and therapy related.
- Agree to supervision whilst practising in the hospice.
- Agree to an appropriate probationary period to establish that the arrangement is working out – both for them and the unit.
- Agree to attend an appropriate induction course and regular workshops.

When working in the hospice, therapists will need to:

- Be insured to practise.
- Be accountable to the doctor in charge of the patient care.
- Cooperate with a supervisor or group of supervisors. This could involve an external supervisor/mentor.
- Discuss within the team whether or not a particular therapy could be helpful generally with the kinds of patients in the unit.
- Observe confidentality about patient related information.

When treating a specific patient the therapist must:

- Obtain informed consent.
- Check the patients up-to-date situation at each visit before approaching them.
- Keep records of each treatment in a place that will be accessible to the doctor in charge of the patient's care.
- Have a means of evaluating the benefit of the therapy to the patient.

© 1995 St Oswald's Hospice

19

Occupational therapy

Jo Bray

Introduction

The role of the occupational therapist in hospice care must be clearly defined and accepted by all members of the inter-disciplinary team, as patients with a progressive illness require more than just physical care: they need to maintain their independence, function and role within the family. The skills of the occupational therapist enable certain aspects of a patient's and carer's life to be assessed, addressing the physical, functional, psychological and social components and also considering the adaptive behaviour, the correction of underlying problems and/or changes in environment, which, together with the skills of the other members of the inter-disciplinary team, maximise independence and quality of life for the dying patient and their carer.

Rehabilitation

Rehabilitation is defined in the Oxford Dictionary as 'to restore to a former condition or status'. Questions must arise as to the appropriateness of this description to the therapy provided and received by patients with a non-curable disease. Dietz suggests that the goal of rehabilitation for people with cancer is to improve the quality of life for a maximum productivity with minimum dependence regardless of life expectancy.[1]

The rehabilitation process for cancer patients can be defined in four stages, and a patient can move between any or all of these stages:

- Preventative rehabilitation – treatment in anticipation of potential disability to lessen severity.
- Restorative rehabilitation – that the patient can be expected to return to premorbid status without significant handicap.
- Supportive rehabilitation – ongoing controlled disease but appropriate rehabilitation can prevent complications which might occur.
- Palliative rehabilitation – progressive disease but appropriate rehabilitation can prevent complications from occurring.

In identifying these four stages the therapist is provided with a realistic treatment approach to facilitate patient-centred goals.

Reed and Sanderson[2] have defined a model of occupation therapy: 'Human Occupations Model', based on a problem-solving approach. The occupational therapist identifies the unique processes, concepts, techniques, concerns and assumptions and ultimately the outcomes of occupational therapy. The focus is

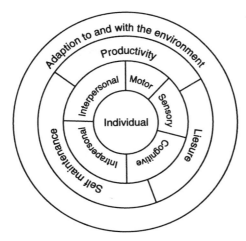

Fig. 19.1 Reed and Sanderson's Human Occupations Model (an adaptation).[3]

that of 'wellness' and is not based on a medical model. A framework is developed focused around the individual and his/her environment and a structured assessment made addressing the individual's 'occupation'. This is any activity requiring the individual's time and energy and using his/her skills, and it has a value (i.e. learned behaviour and a belief in something). These occupations are related to 'self maintenance', 'productivity' and 'leisure'. The individual must have a level of competence and the components required to carry out these 'occupations', the components being motor, sensory, cognitive, intrapersonal and interpersonal.

Definitions

Performance components

Motor skills – the level, quality and/or degree of range of motion, gross muscle strength, muscle tone, endurance, fine motor skills and functional use.

Sensory skills – refers to skills and performance in perceiving and differentiating external and internal stimuli.

Cognitive skills – the level, quality and/or degree of comprehension, communication, concentration, problem solving, time management, conceptualisation, integration of learning, judgement and time/place/person orientation.

Intrapersonal skills – the level, quality and/or degree of self identity, self concept and coping skills.

Interpersonal skills – the level, quality and/or degree of dyadic and group interaction skills.

Occupational components

Self-maintenance occupations – those activities or tasks which are done routinely to maintain the person's health and well-being in the environment such as dressing or eating.

Productivity occupations – those activities or tasks which are done to enable the person to provide support to the self, family and society.

Leisure occupations – those activities or tasks done for the enjoyment and renewal that the activity or task brings to the person. They may contribute to the promotion of health and well-being.

In utilising this model of occupational therapy, the occupational therapist uses a 'client–centred', 'problem–oriented' approach, complementing the hospice philosophy in improving the individual's quality of life.

Motor skills

For many patients this component is dependent on muscle wastage or weakness which may be due to weight loss or weight gain. The result of this on the patient is loss of range of movement, ease of transfers or general mobility and fatigue. The early introduction and supply of equipment (for example a bath board) may maintain the patient's independence, thus giving a positive experience. With their decline, they may require additional support from a carer or professional. If equipment is supplied in the latter stages of decline, it is perceived as a reinforcement of that decline and viewed negatively.

A similar comparison can be made to the use and supply of wheelchairs. Owing to reduced energy levels and fatigue a patient may benefit from the supply of a wheelchair for long distance, outdoor use, however sufficiently mobile they may be around their own home and garden. Positive experiences and pleasurable memories all ease the acceptance when the patient is limited further.

General advice can be given by the occupational therapist regarding energy conservation, the staging of activities throughout the day, limiting stair climbing, sitting while carrying out activities, noting heights of surfaces for transfers and frequency. Alternative techniques of carrying out activity can be taught.

It is important to establish what the priority is for the patient, getting them to set the goals, accepting the focus to the important activities and recognising help from others in completing less important tasks.

Sensory

Patients experience a wide degree and variety of pain, and often a patient's pain can be described as 'total pain', the focus of which may not be a physical sensation. It is important to recognise the whole concept of pain when implementing occupational therapy assessment and treatment programmes and its influence over the 'occupations' and activity. This may mean coordinating the timing of treatment sessions prior to administering of medication to facilitate optimal functioning.

Patients may have distorted or loss of sensation as a result of tumour growth on a direct nerve, fibrosing of tissues or it may be induced medically for pain control.

Advice and supply of equipment may be necessary to prevent accidental damage, for example patients with upper limb secondary lymphoedema, within the kitchen.

Loss of sensation decreases the patient's awareness of the development of pressure sores, and the pain from such sores can have a dramatic effect on a person's well-being. The supply of appropriate cushions and mattresses is essential to the prevention of pressure sores. Occupational therapists have a wealth of knowledge on a wide range of pressure-relieving cushions.

Cognitive

Cognitive impairment may be a direct result from tumour growth within the brain or from secondaries. It may be as a result of side-effects from medication or dramatic effects of fatigue. Those with direct tumour growth require a sound neurological approach to a treatment programme to be implemented by the occupational therapist.

All aspects of communication, comprehension, concentration and organisational skills need to be assessed by the occupational therapist as these are vital to the functioning of any 'occupations'.

It is essential that the occupational therapist conveys to the patient that he or she has unpressured, quality time to give. They must have highly developed communication skills in order that the patient communicates his/her goals and not those of the therapist.

Intrapersonal

Poor self image can drastically inhibit the functioning of an individual with the 'occupations'/activities required in life. Feelings of anxiety and stress should be recognised and relaxation programmes taught to develop coping mechanisms to deal with such feelings in everyday life.

Patients whose 'occupational' performance is affected by their intrapersonal skills may need psychological support from trained professionals. In such situations occupational therapists should refer on to appropriate agencies.

Goal setting has the positive benefit of facilitating patients' involvement and subsequent control over their lives. Recognition should also be made to significant life events as these themselves can become the focus and goal to so many patients.

Interpersonal

The focus of many patients' lives becomes disease orientated. Patients lose control, lose their roles and, in turn, self confidence, self worth and respect. Patients should therefore be encouraged to set goals to facilitate some control within their lives and to increase their motivation and positive feelings of self worth in order to be valued as an individual. The use of a structured programme of activity within a hospice day care centre can constructively use groupwork to enhance these positive feelings.

Having addressed the performance components or skills required by the individual, one then focuses on the 'occupational' components, the activities in routine daily life.

Self maintenance

This involves the skills of personal activities of daily living: washing, bathing, dressing and toileting, and domestic activities: shopping, cooking, laundry, cleaning and general household duties.

With consideration to the performance components, the occupational therapist assesses the patient's abilities to carry out these tasks of self maintenance. The focus of assessment should not be limited to performance outcomes/ achievements but to those tasks that are of significance to the patient and how these can be achieved. The occupational therapist will correct underlying problems, teach alternative methods or supply appropriate equipment in order to maintain independence. Those activities that are not of significance to achieve independence may be carried out by a carer or professional, or they may assist the patient with the task. It is important that where possible the patient has the choice and thus can maintain control for as long as is feasible.

Productivity

Throughout all stages of a patient's decline it is important for the patient to feel productive. Many may have lost employment, their role associated with this, their income, their role as a parent, husband, wife or family member, the focus of their lives being disease-led. Becoming a patient, an invalid, can lead to feelings of passivity and dependency.

An occupational therapist can work with a patient and their limited functional ability to provide some structure or new role to encourage productivity. This could range from constructively filling free time from the loss of employment to exchanging family roles of the 'bread winner' to 'housekeeper' or, if energy levels are severely limited, coordinating the shopping list for a home carer.

Leisure

Leisure covers the activities from which a patient derives pleasure. It is important for our psychological well-being that some part of every day we gain pleasure or enjoyment from something. It is, therefore, even more important for our patients, and in assessing patients' 'occupational components' care must be taken to address this area, ensuring that energy levels and functional abilities still allow pleasurable experiences. As a patient declines these are often small requests, but they have immense significance to the patient. It is important to recognise these and, where possible realistically, that they be achieved.

Conclusion

If the future commitment of palliative care is to address comprehensively the quality of life of patients with maximum productivity and minimum dependency, then occupational therapists are essential members of the multi-disciplinary team, in order to maximise patients' independence and functional level within the limits of their declining health.

References

1. Dietz JH. *Rehabilitation oncology*. New York: John Wiley, 1981.
2. Reed K, Sanderson S. *Concepts of occupational therapy*, 2nd edn. Baltimore: Williams & Wilkins, 1988.
3. Hagedorn K. *Occupational therapy: foundations for practice models, frames of reference and core skills*. London: Churchill Livingstone, 1992; 64–7.

Further reading

Hockley J. Rehabilitation in palliative care – are we asking the impossible? *Palliative Med* 1993, 7: 9–15.
Turner A, Foster M, Johnson SE, eds. *Occupational therapy and physical dysfunction: principles, skills and practice*, 3rd edn. London: Churchill Livingstone, 1992.

20

A–Z of creative therapies

Jo Bray

Introduction

This chapter is written for professionals working in day care centres. It can be used as a resource to be referred to as the need arises or as an introduction to the fascinating and rewarding application of purposeful activity within a structured day care programme.

Activity programmes

The activity programme within day care provides patients with an awareness of future events. It enables staff to plan and prepare groups, which is vital for the success of any activity. The programme should provide a comprehensive range of activities, skills, hobbies and interests to ensure that the diversity of human needs are met.

A planned activity programme far exceeds the limits of diversional therapy which so often isolates the patient. It encompasses the ethos of group work and group dynamics with a defined structure and purpose. It enables critical examination, to reflect on past programmes of activity and enable re-evaluation of aims and objectives for future programmes, thus avoiding activities becoming routine with the inevitable institutionalisation of staff and patients. It provides an opportunity for generation of new ideas and concepts and can be a means of motivating staff.

Aims of day care

Whilst recognising that not all day care units have the same client group or needs, aims should be clearly identified in order that evaluation and development of service provision can be undertaken.

This is a list of some areas that may be considered:

- For patients to be able to identify with a peer group;
- To offer respite for carers;
- To reduce patient isolation;
- To facilitate positive feelings of self worth, confidence, esteem, motivation and success;
- To provide stimulation for patient;
- To enable patients to recapture and relearn diverse skills whilst providing enjoyment and fun;
- To recognise patients' individuality and provide a range of services/activities that address the patients' holistic needs.

Alcohol

Alcohol is recognised as an appetite stimulant and should be offered as pre-lunch drinks.

There is a cost implication and this must be budgeted for and, for safety reasons, the alcohol must be stored in a locked cupboard.

Aromatherapy – *See* Complementary therapies

Art

Art is often something that many patients have not experienced since school days, and so this may rekindle either fond memories or feelings of fear and failure. However, art used with a purpose, structure and support can be invaluable to those less able to express themselves verbally.

Patients may feel very dissatisfied with their attempts to produce artistic-looking pictures, so it is important to have a good introduction with the use of a theme, topic, word or words. Patients should then be made aware that they will have an opportunity to explain or 'think through' their picture and share their thoughts with the group, removing the emphasis from artistic quality and highlighting picture individuality.

Barbecues

Many hospices are situated in splendid grounds, and, if fortunate to have access to them, these should be utilised to a maximum. Barbecues can provide a social activity whilst enjoying the gardens. They have often proved most beneficial to patients with poor appetites as they provide an interest in food; the smell alone tempting many patients.

Obviously, due to food hygiene regulations, those handling and cooking the food must meet the requirements,[1] hence close links should be established with the kitchen staff. Vegetarian requirements should also be considered.

Even when the 'British summer' lets you down, it is well worth braving the elements to cook outdoors and serve the food inside.

Beauty therapy

Patients who are tired, have low energy levels, poor motivation and concentration and are often depressed, pay little attention to their physical appearance. Touch is a powerful medium in itself, as is receiving time and attention from another. Patients through their disease process often look pale and ill, and beauty therapy can enable them to feel more positive about themselves, thus boosting their self confidence and self esteem.

Beauty therapy should not be viewed as a female activity, as men can gain many benefits from a manicure or neck and shoulder massage.

A variety of agencies and staff, for example the British Red Cross, have trained beauty therapists who provide services free. Volunteers may have specific skills in this area. Establishing links with local branches of *The Body Shop* can prove beneficial, with regular talks, make-overs and hand massages. Local department stores may offer one-off sessions providing make-up demonstrations and then making up each patient. A camera can often prove to be beneficial on such occasions.

Birthdays

Celebrating patients' birthdays on their day of attendance enables other patients to participate in and contribute to a special activity. A birthday cake and secretly signed card and photographs of the day make for a memorable event.

Chaplains

Chaplains have a vital role within day care and for the spiritual care of patients and staff. However, there is a fine balance between those who wish to access the chaplains and those who have no specific feelings to do so. A suggestion would be to regularly invite a chaplain to lunch; patients can then seek to use the chaplain in the way they so wish. It is ideal if significant religious events incorporated into the planned day care programme are also associated with the chaplain's visit. This has advantages for the patients and the chaplains in getting to know each other, and perhaps the chaplain could stay and join in with activities after lunch, such as art groups, and subsequent discussions.

Chiropody

Many elderly people cannot physically care for their feet, nor have access to a chiropody service in the community, nor be able to afford it privately.

Day care should negotiate special rates with a local mobile chiropodist who will visit patients every 6–8 weeks. This can be worked so that the chiropodist visits on a rotational basis, but is in the hospice weekly, ensuring that in-patients will also have access to the service. This guarantee of a large number of patients may help in the negotiation of cheaper rates.

Christmas

Where do you start?!

So many patients involved in day care will celebrate their last Christmas, and so for many it becomes an important focus. Hence the need to make as much of the event and the build-up to it as is reasonably possible. Everyone has their own ideas of celebrating Christmas.

The following is a list of some Christmas activities:

• Print and make Christmas cards;
• Make and decorate Christmas cakes;
• Make chocolates and truffles;
• Make a Christmas collage;
• Reminiscence groups of Christmas traditions;

- Christmas pictionary;
- Make Christmas decorations for fund-raising tree;
- Visit local supermarket and purchase small items;
- Pot pourri – spicy Christmas;
- Orange pomanders;
- Make small gifts;
- Christmas party lunch – every patient having a Christmas present;
- Local primary school entertainment following lunch, e.g. songs, reading, plays.

Cocktail tasting (*see also* Dietician)

Sadly, and to the disappointment of many patients, this contains very little, or no, alcohol! The aim of a cocktail tasting session is to address the dietary needs of the group and complement talks from dieticians.

The cocktails are made from recipes/cocktails from the high-protein, high-nutrient, dietary supplements. Recipe sheets are available from the companies who produce the supplements, also available are free samples which could be used in making up the cocktails or given to patients by contacting the regional representative for the area.

This raises patient awareness as to what products are available, and the variety of uses of the product, which makes them more interesting than 'just a drink from a carton'!

Collage

A wide range of topics can be used to create a collage; however, there must be sufficient space to display the end result.

Collage is open to any artistic talent, or lack of it! However, strong glue is a necessity. It can bring together work of all day care patients. It can also be an advocate for the work of day care, or display in the hospice – the reception area or other well-used area is ideal.

The following is a list of suggested themes for collage:

- Items to be taken to a desert island;
- A day care tree, every patient contributing a leaf;
- Using a sea, beach or shore-line theme, ask what the patients would wish to be in the collage, and why;
- The seasons – an ongoing project throughout the year;
- Christmas: a favourite association, a nativity scene, a Christmas carol, an Advent calendar.

The list is endless with careful thought and imagination.

Communication groups

Communication is vital to us all; however, when any of us are temporarily depressed, anxious or low in self esteem, our relationship with others is affected, which often results in a tendency to become withdrawn, over-demanding or unreceptive. Patients attending day care can have good family support but be over protected, often becoming withdrawn and lacking in confidence and initiating conversation. Some are socially isolated, their regular communication being with professionals from community-based support. The latter can tend to want to talk at someone, with their responses to effective communication limited, as are their listening skills.

Groups could be run at the start of the day to facilitate communication amongst the day care patients, the aim being for patients to speak to the patient either side of them. This is especially beneficial when integrating new patients or new in-patients. (This can also reduce the development of 'special bonds' – 'I always sit in that chair next to Nellie', etc.)

See Group Dynamics for running groups, and Quizzes for ideas of content/ material.

Complementary therapies

There are many therapies and healing arts available, offering a wide variety of approaches to health and well-being, many of them complementary to orthodox medicine. Some are more well known than others and they can vary in availability and accessibility. Some complementary therapies are practised to clear standards of competency and performance, with full professional indemnity, third party liability, a code of ethics, records and referral to other professionals including doctors when appropriate, while others are not. There are guidelines on therapists' training and accreditation and the Institute for Complementary Medicine is compiling a British Register of Complementary Practitioners.[2]

When establishing complementary therapies in the day care programme, consultation should be sought from the medical director of the centre.

For a more detailed account of each specific therapy, further reading is recommended.

Cookery

Cookery can be of interest to both men and women and it can be an appetite stimulant to those with poor nutritional states. However, for those with altered taste and smell the mere suggestion of cookery can have negative results.

It is important to have good links with the kitchen staff for the supply of, or access to central purchasing of, ingredients and, where necessary, the cooking of the end result.

Minimal handling of food should take place, and one must ensure that patients receive their own end product. This can be done by writing each patient's name on greaseproof paper, e.g. in lining a cake tin for a Christmas cake or baking sheet for biscuits.

If patients wish to take the products home, then staff should ensure in their planning that there is sufficient time for cooking.

If patients have assisted in the making of a product then this will not meet the food hygiene regulations and, therefore, cannot be sold.[3]

Examples

Christmas cakes. Individual cakes can be made using a 15-oz lined tin can.

Mixture sufficient for an 8-inch cake will make four of the above size, cooked at the temperature stated in the recipe and usually for the same length of time. They can then be decorated using fondant icing.

For day care to establish the choice of recipe, a Christmas reminiscence group can be based around this theme, with amazing storytelling of times gone by.

The cake provides an ideal gift for those going to stay with family over Christmas, or for grandchildren. For those living alone it provides a means of social contact with neighbours or community support agencies, who will have a piece of cake with their patient.

Biscuits. These can be made throughout the year. Kitchen staff prepare the mixture, patients roll out and cut shapes. A suitable recipe requires 6 minutes cooking time, which ensures all patients can take home their own biscuits.

Chocolates and truffles. These can be made in day care and centres with no kitchen support. A slow cooker is the ideal solution and enables chocolate to be melted with the least risk to patients. (Slow cookers could be borrowed from staff members – however make sure they meet the centre's electrical appliance regulations – or they could be purchased.) Four to six patients can assist in the preparation of a mixture, which can be divided between them to shape. Prepared boxes could make these a very presentable gift, especially at Christmas or Easter.

Chocolate eggs. Using chocolate shell moulds, melted chocolate can be poured into the moulds and left to dry. More adventurous patients or volunteers/staff can ice names on the eggs. Very successful for grandchildren.

Cookery book

Each patient makes a contribution to the centre's cookery book, giving their favourite meal, snack or recipe with the reason or story behind their choice. These can be collated and, when well presented, can be sold at sales of work or fetes.

Creative challenge

The aim of this is to facilitate group interaction and provide stimulation and team work. Boxes containing identical items of, for example, card, fabric, string, ribbon, coat hangers, toilet roll tubes, plastic bottles and imagination, are provided for participating groups. Each group is given clear instruction that the object of the exercise is to make/construct something from the items in the box, with a time limit of 30 minutes. The idea is not to produce a masterpiece or quality work. It is about working together as a team and producing something as an end result. This can prove very successful as two groups can create things poles apart, e.g. a puppet theatre and mobile to a game and boat from the same contents. It may sound odd, but this activity really gets people working together and is especially useful when new patients attend, as they are readily made a part of the group.

Crosswords

Knowing the client group is a prerequisite of this activity.

Activity method

Select a crossword from a newspaper, magazine or quiz book that would be suitable for your client group. Transfer the grid on to a large poster. Having opposing teams adds to the challenge and competitiveness, and by using different coloured pens each team's answers can easily be identified. Completing crosswords as a team effort affords individuals who have failing eyesight, memory loss or poor concentration the satisfaction of participating in an activity that gave them pleasure.

Dietary needs in day care

Where possible a choice of food should be available at lunch time, ranging from a three-course meal to snacks and sandwiches. A ready supply of hot and cold drinks should also be available if required. Pre-lunch alcoholic drinks may help as an appetite stimulant. Chocolate biscuits with morning coffee, cakes with afternoon tea, sweets, mints and chocolates after lunch all add to the calorific intake that so many patients lack.

Special dietary needs, e.g. diabetic, soft liquidised diet should also be available. Encouraging dietary intake with special thematic days and seasonal events, e.g. cream teas in summer, choc ices or popcorn whilst watching videos and planning visits to pubs or restaurants so that patients' needs are catered for, ensures that patients' nutritional requirements are also met.

Dietitians

Not many centres are fortunate to have the skills of a dietitian as a member of the multi-disciplinary team, so one has to try to establish links locally. Hospital or community dietitians may give a half hour talk, give advice over the telephone or provide handouts. Prepared literature may be a means of 'doing it yourself'.

Some of the companies who manufacture the high-protein, nutrition supplements also produce good leaflets and recipes. Sales representatives may be willing to give talks, but the focus may be on the supplements and not addressing the question of 'What do I eat if I'm not feeling hungry?'

Discussion groups

With careful thought and preparation and the appropriate professional skills, there is no reason why discussion groups should not take place within day care.

Patients should not be forced to talk openly about their disease, as many will be at different stages of working through their current problems, futures and prognosis. 'Safe' topics should be used, e.g. current affairs, music, films, theatre, TV, the Royal Family and reminiscence. In this situation, it is advisable to have skilled members of staff who, following these discussions, have access to support themselves. It would certainly be advisable to have two members of staff when running such a group.

Diversional therapy

Diversional therapy should never be confused with occupational therapy nor purposeful activity. By definition, diversion is an occupation of the mind, whereas purposeful activity has a well-defined structure with aims, patient-set goals and an evaluation strategy.

Entertainment

Entertainment from outside agencies is always well received within day care. The obvious choice is 'Music in Hospitals', who, although they charge a fee, constantly provide a wide variety of professional musicians of a high standard. Staff may have contacts locally, but this often causes problems in seeking entertainment as the participants often work during the day. Local theatres, ballet or orchestras can be very charitable to day care. Schools provide excellent entertainment, especially around Christmas, but one must remember that this needs to be in term time.

Entertainment should be limited as most patients' concentration span is usually 30–45 minutes. If in-patients have joined in the entertainment, careful attention should be given as they may not tolerate the duration of the performance and, therefore, may benefit from sitting near the exit (as may those with poor bladder and bowel control). It is far easier to extend a performance that is being well received than attempt to rectify a bored, sleepy group of patients, when the positive gain could have been lost and outweighed by gloom!

Exercise – 'keep fit'

This should be more appropriately titled 'keep things going'!

Where possible exercises should be conducted by a qualified physiotherapist as they have the expert knowledge of the range of movement, of specific muscle groups that should be maintained, as well as functional abilities and capabilities of the patients. They can recognise patients' weaknesses and deterioration and structure sessions appropriately. However, a half-hour keep fit session enables one physiotherapist to have contact with the whole group of patients and can identify those requiring individual treatment programmes.

Keep fit can be the ideal way to start the afternoon as it 'bucks things up' after lunch and the natural sleepy time as a result of a full stomach!

Flower arranging

Flower arranging may be viewed as a female activity; however, with encouragement and a light-hearted approach, many men will also join in such an activity. It can be particularly useful at Christmas time, making table and door decorations. Patients make one for themselves to take home at no charge, but also make an additional one which can be sold amongst the staff of the centre.

Most of the foliage for flower decorations can be collected from the centre's grounds or staff gardens. With minimal cost for oasis, dishes and ribbon, an income can be easily generated, thus enabling the purchase of a small Christmas present for each patient or treats for the Christmas lunches.

Many volunteers may be interested and assist with the flower arranging sessions. Contacts may also be made locally with flower clubs who may also give demonstrations.

Fun

Day care, although having sad times at the loss of members, should on the whole be a place of pleasure, enjoyment and fun. It should not be forced nor inflicted upon patients. A well-balanced team of staff and volunteers with good skill mix, motivation and enthusiasm has the means to create such an environment.

In so doing, patients look forward to attending the centre and will often make the effort, when perhaps they are not feeling at their best, but know by attending they will feel better: 'It's taken my mind off it!'.

Staff should regularly evaluate day care activities in order to dispel complacency.

Games on the lawn

On the occasions that the British weather allows, it is invaluable to maximise the centre's grounds by using a wide selection of lawn games, or just sitting and watching others whilst enjoying a cream tea. This is especially beneficial for housebound/wheelchair users as it expands their horizons and pleasures when attending the day centre.

Gaming

Gaming invariably increases interest and tends to help patients loosen up and become more fully involved. The fact that it is a game gives participants permission to be silly and allows laughter and enjoyment where this might otherwise be considered inappropriate. For this reason a game can be an effective way to start sessions, loosening up attitudes and encouraging active engagement.

Goal setting

The setting of goals, however small or large, provides structure, purpose and aims to activity. They should be realistic, achievable within the time limit and, where necessary, structured to the individual's needs. Initially, goals should be simplistic so that satisfaction and success are achieved. Positive feedback and encouragement should be given.

In achieving goals, patients' roles of passivity and dependency are reduced, and confidence, self esteem and self worth are enhanced.

Group dynamics

A minimum group should be four to six patients, with the simplistic aim of establishing a rapport: patient to patient and patient to staff. Patients are brought together from a wide variety of backgrounds, and within a group each member is of equal status – 'a participant'. The success of a group is due to the contribution of all members.

Setting simple rules to the group creates safe boundaries for the participants.

The positive aims of group work are to reduce isolation, increase confidence and self esteem, facilitate stimulation, and in turn, motivation. Other aims are to develop concentration, interaction and team work, but ultimately to provoke interest and fun.

Hairdressing

Hairdressing can be provided from a variety of sources to complement the activity programme. Gifted staff or volunteers may utilise skills on an *ad hoc* basis. More formal sessions may be offered by a skilled hairdresser, maybe volunteers with training, or by establishing links locally with a voluntary hairdressing service. A mobile hairdresser may negotiate cheaper rates for the patients if a regular morning is allocated to the centre.

See also Beauty therapy.

Health and safety

Lifting and handling is a vast subject; however, all staff and volunteers require mandatory training to comply with the health and safety rules and regulations and those set out by the EC Directive.[4]

Volunteers in day care may not directly be handling patients but still require knowledge of how to assist a patient, and to recognise their own limitations and the necessity for staff assistance. This is vital to those centres using volunteer drivers to transport patients. Those centres making risk assessment of their patients' handling needs must ensure that these are accessible and available to volunteers and staff and are regularly updated to meet the patients' changing needs.

Food handling and hygiene is equally a vast area, but one which must also be taken seriously.[5] Hence food handled by patients can only be consumed by them. Where possible, maximum effort must be made to ensure patients receive their own handled food. Under no circumstances can any foods prepared by staff/volunteers without the food-handling certificate, or by patients, be sold.[6]

Hobbies

Many of the activities should be based on patients' past hobbies or interests that they can no longer achieve outside the centre and should be of a wide and diverse selection. New hobbies should be available for everyone to experience and develop new skills. Regionally patients may have specific hobbies or interests. Outside speakers may provide an excellent means of patients accessing more physically demanding hobbies, e.g. travel, walking/rambling, bird watching.

Horticulture

Most patients have, at some period in their lives, had access to a garden or taken an interest in plants. Many patients because of their disease do not have sufficient energy to maintain their own gardens; however, they may still have vast knowledge and experience that can be utilised to recapture pleasure they previously experienced.

Creating gardening into a 'desk-top' activity eliminates the physical strain. Producing potted plants, cuttings, herb gardens, hanging baskets, tubs and grow bags with tomatoes can all be achieved in a centre with no actual garden.

Demonstrations from local garden centres can provide excellent stimulation. Income generation can be well utilised from such projects, for example making up hanging baskets and selling them on to staff within the centre. (A demonstration from the local garden centre can ensure a more professional looking hanging basket.)

Obviously, this activity can be developed further in centres with specific garden areas and greenhouses. Making access easy for wheelchair users and raising flower beds are obvious musts if this activity is to be fully utilised by all patients.

Gardening is such a common theme for many, but for those with a specific interest in the area then the enjoyment, stimulation and sharing of knowledge creates many pleasurable memories.

Imaginative staff

Yes!

A dynamic activity programme requires effort, imagination and support from staff who are constantly seeking new ideas and regularly question the structure process and outcome. Be brave in trying new ideas and be honest in admitting success and failure.

Income generation

Day care centres' and materials' budgets are structured in a variety of ways, from no budget to those that are well funded. However, it is true to say that most are charitable organisations with limited finances.

Day care activity should not be seen as a means of income generation to any centre; this should be a secondary gain from the activity. Patients do receive great satisfaction from feeling that they have contributed something to the centre in return for the care they receive. Carefully managed projects can contribute greatly to a day care budget, e.g. printing (tickets, invitations, letter-headed stationery, birthday, Easter and Christmas cards), horticulture (hanging baskets, herb gardens, cuttings, Christmas table and door decorations), sales of work.

Projects using materials which are scrap or waste or have been donated obviously maximise the profit.

Jigsaws

The application of group dynamics and goal achievement should be utilised to facilitate a more imaginative approach to the use and purpose of jigsaws within a day care activity programme.

Jigsaws can facilitate team work, competitive spirit, concentration, cognition and dexterity.

Keep fit (*see* Exercise)

Library

Most patients cannot get to their local library; however they have plenty of time to read which, although requiring concentration, requires little energy.

The British Red Cross society, or other local agency, can offer an actual library service, including large print books. Many staff and volunteers will donate a collection of paperbacks for day care to offer its own informal library service, which could also include magazines.

For those who have poor eyesight but who have previously enjoyed reading, day care could have a talking book machine for patients to try. If this is successful then arrangements could be made for the patient to have their own machine. For patients who do not have carers to re-order books/tapes then this could be something taken on by day care. Grants could be sought for those unable to fund the annual hire. Contacts could also be established for a local talking newspaper.

Lunches out

Income generated from projects such as hanging baskets, Christmas decorations, etc., can enable day care to take all patients out for lunch (hence no pressure is imposed on those with limited finances).

A pre-visit to the venue or telephone contact is vital to ensure good access facilities and amenities especially for wheelchair users. The pub/restaurant should be well lit with good floor surfaces, avoiding scattered rugs/carpets or several floor levels with occasional steps.

Some places offer half portions or OAP menus which are ideal for patients as they are not faced with a huge meal.

It is worth keeping a watch for local pubs/restaurants which close for refurbishment: prior to re-opening they often have 'dry runs' when they are closed to the general public but require customers to enable the restaurant to run at full capacity. We have been guests at such occasions with great success. It is often a free meal (drinks not included), but patients gain great satisfaction from being 'special guests' and giving their opinions on the food, decor and service. This often means contacting people senior to the pub/restaurant manager, e.g. the retail operation manager.

Lunch guests

At lunch patients can be left to socialise amongst themselves; staff are not normally present. If the communication group in the morning has served its purpose then the 'ice' has been broken and the group of patients should be chatting freely amongst themselves. Lunch time is the patients' only real time to socialise freely and recognise that they are not the only person 'going through this'.

On a rotational basis, each day of day care has a lunch guest once a month. The guests are people patients should be aware of within the more extended day care team, knowing their services are accessible if requested, e.g. matron/manager, chaplain, social worker, home care team, doctor. Patients discuss whatever they wish with the member of staff, which may be kept at a social level or taken further.

This may also be extended to include the ward sister, nursing staff and team leaders as well as the voluntary services coordinator

Maslow's hierarchy of needs

Animals and humans are driven to act in order to satisfy their own needs; these needs can be arranged in a hierarchical order. The more simplistic needs have to be met in order to strive towards the more complex needs to reach self fulfilment (self actualisation).[7]

Physical needs

Those of food, water, shelter – the basic physical requirements to life.

Day care can provide equipment for comfort and conserving energy; offer advice and facilitate maximum independence of activities or daily living, relief from physical pain and other symptoms.

Safety needs

Those of order and stability within one's self and in relationships with others.

Day care can provide support and advise family; reduce tension at home; alleviate anxiety and provide advice on management of stress.

Esteem

The needs of self respect, feelings of success, sense of belonging and love.

Day care can provide and facilitate emotional, psychological and spiritual support; alleviate over-introspection, boredom and anxiety (which compounds suffering); enable patients to give as well as receive; introduce tasks that are of value and worth to others; encourage self expression, creativity, humour; enable patients to develop social contacts.

Self actualisation

Those feelings of competence, achievement and success.

Day care can actively involve patients in decision making to achieve their own goals; demonstrate to patients their own strengths and capabilities; provide opportunities for broadening experiences and interests while horizons are narrowing.

Maslow (1954) defines abnormality as 'anything that frustrates or blocks or denies the essential nature of man ... anything that disturbs or frustrates or twists the course of actualisation'.[8] Patients with a limited prognosis should be facilitated to reach a position from which self actualisation becomes a possibility.

Memorial service

The memory of, and respect given to, a patient who has died is important to those in the group, not only for the individual memories of the patient but also for those present in the group to know they too will receive recognition.

The whole area of loss and bereavement at the patient level is something which needs careful thought as to what will work in the centre and what is available to do so. This may range from patients signing a sympathy card sent to the next of kin, to the chaplain conducting a more formal memorial service. However, it is an area which should not be forgotten nor avoided.

The day centre manager must establish some means of observing and recognising the emotions of the staff and volunteers. There are occasions, even with the highest quality staff and volunteers, when emotions are stirred and appropriate support should be available. It should be stressed that this is not a failure or weakness on anyone's part (unless this is atypical and more appropriate action should then be taken).

Manicures

(*See* Beauty therapy)

Music in hospitals

'Music in Hospitals' is a charitable organisation offering a wide range of professional entertainment, all of which are extremely sensitive to the needs of patients. There is a charge and pre-booking is necessary.

See also Entertainment.

Music

Making music or listening to music are activities which contain a strong emotional element. Styles of music can facilitate different moods or emotions. Taste in music is subjective, therefore a range of music should be available and sensitivity shown to patients' choice or dislikes.

Listening to music can be used as a specific activity, as it may improve awareness of the environment and discrimination between tones and emotions.

Making music can be a simple activity using a variety of objects or parts of the body to establish rhythmic sounds.

Background music throughout lunch can prevent the development of long silences and pressure to communicate, and can facilitate a relaxing period following lunch.

Newsletter

Centres may produce a weekly newsletter, which facilitates cross reference of the patients attending different days of the week, produced by staff.

Quarterly newsletters may be produced by patients, writing reviews of past events or comments and feelings of their perceived view of day care and the reality.

Both of these may be beneficial in the community, especially those with patients' views, as they may encourage new patients to attend day care.

Notice board

The notice board should be accessible to patients and be informative, eye-catching, stimulating and relevant to up and coming events. It should be changed regularly and, with photos, can be a log of past events. Items displayed should be large enough for patients to read.

It may be helpful to have photographs of staff displayed as a 'Who's Who,' and all the above comments apply.

Operational policy

Every day care centre should have an operational policy. This document refers to the smooth running of the day-to-day procedures, stating what is required and how it will be achieved.

The policy should include:

• Physical amenities;
• Staffing;
• Service provision;
• Referral and discharge procedure.

Outings

Attending day care for many patients may be their only means of getting out. Outings should be well planned as preparation is vital to the smooth running and ensuring maximum benefit to patients. (Pre-visits, considering wheelchair access, amenities and facilities may be necessary.)

With the cold and wet weather of winter many patients are content in attending day care. However, with the onset of sunny, warmer days from late March to September, outings enhance the patient's day.

Because patients tire easily, distances travelled should be kept to a minimum. Wheelchairs should be offered to all, ensuring sufficient staff and volunteers are available. Nursing staff should not wear uniform. A prepared bag, including vomit bowls, damp sponge/cloths, tissues, etc., should be taken. A camera is vital. Outings should occur regularly and, where possible, be of the patients' choice.

A prepared policy and procedure should be in operation regarding patient safety and action taken accordingly in the event of an incident or emergency.

Transport contacts could be established locally for those centres without their own mini bus (local education departments, community and social services or voluntary organisations may be useful suppliers).

Papier mâché

Papier mâché can be used successfully in making a variety of shapes and sizes of bowls and may be linked to theme days.

Cling film is used to cover any bowl or plate and a layer of newspaper strips soaked in water is then applied to cover the cling film. Repeated layers of newspaper strips are then applied, using wallpaper paste as an adhesive. At least eight layers of paper should be applied, but more will give the bowl additional strength.

After being left to dry, the bowl can be coated with varnish and later emulsioned. Various techniques can be used to decorate the end result: stencilling, sponging, etc.

Some of the stages may require staff in order to successfully complete.

Patchwork

Patchwork can be used for successful projects such as collage, wall hangings, cushions or group projects to present to charities or for raffles.

Older patients may lack the dexterity to produce the card-mounted patches, although volunteers can assist in the preparation. Patients, if they are able, pin and tack the patches on to Vyleen, which is then machine stitched to finish off, a willing seamstress/volunteer could come to the rescue yet again!

If patchwork cushions are to be used in the centre or sold for funds. Then the fabric and cushion pads used must meet the fire safety regulations.

Pet therapy

It is a long-established fact that animals have a therapeutic value to humans. How this is practically included within the day care programme is subject to local interpretation, and can be provided by a resident budgie, fish or cat to regular visits from 'pat dogs'.

Many patients throughout their lives have owned an animal and the pleasure from their contact is evident almost instantly.

Care, however, must be taken with patients who are apprehensive or sensitive to animals. Amazingly, animals often are aware of this and respond accordingly, which results in a positive response from patients.

Philosophy of care

We recognise that all too often health care assigns sick and dying persons a role of passivity and dependency. We believe in valuing our patients' individuality and enabling the patient towards self fulfilment and self actualisation.

We believe day care should provide patients with a stimulating and enjoyable day, and our care should be based on a sound therapeutic framework within which activities are selected for a specific purpose and graded to suit a patient's particular needs, thereby promoting confidence and self-worth.

We believe our primary aim is to relieve isolation/loneliness by encouraging communication and identity within a peer group, and secondly to provide respite for carers.

Day Care Philosophy
Warran Pearl Marie Curie Centre 1993

Photograph frames

Photo frames, using pre-cut padded material, can be glued and finished by any member of day care, with or without any craft skills. They can provide excellent gifts or, with a photograph, reinforce a positive experience or memorable event.

Photographs

A camera is a must for any day care, as so many families may neglect to take regular photos of their loved ones. A camera can capture so many of the fun times, a special smile, a visit to the hairdresser, the list is endless. Patients regularly request reprints for themselves or for their families.

For those day centres attached to in-patient units, photographs can be of immense value to bereaved relatives in associating pleasurable memories of their loved ones and may be of benefit if given at the time of collecting the death certificate.

Pot pourri

For those centres with gardens, fresh flowers and shrubs can be collected, layered between tissue paper and left to dry. Then, following set recipes for pot pourri, these can be made into various aromas.

The procedure may take a few sessions over a period of time before being bagged and sold. More interesting presentations can include coloured layers in unusual shaped jam jars, covered with a lace top, or in papier mâché bowls. Cling film placed over the whole bowl shrinks when heated with a hair dryer resulting in a smooth, professional finish.

Pottery

Pottery has been described by some as the means of taking control of the essence of life in your hands. However, it is a pleasurable activity that most patients will participate in. For a more formal approach, a pottery instructor can be used on a sessional basis or links established with local adult education services. Volunteers may have hidden talents, or using pottery books may help staff in a more do it yourself approach.

Self-hardening clay, which dries naturally, can now be purchased from craft suppliers, hence no kiln is required.

Printing

The use of a second-hand Adana printing press can be of immense value in providing people with a stimulating activity. Printing presses and a variety of type can be brought from occupational therapy departments at a cheap price (these are often no longer used due to the reduced length of stay of patients in hospitals).

Local printing companies produce waste card that can readily be utilised to produce birthday, Easter, Christmas and thank-you cards. A guillotine can be a good investment to produce a professional looking card, the final touches added by printing an appropriate message.

Birthday and Christmas cards can be recycled or designed with simple shapes from coloured paper (pre-prepared by volunteers).

The printing of Christmas cards can be a great source of income generation to day care; however, packs of cards have to be rationed as supply does not meet demand.

Questioning

Regular questions must be asked by, and of the team, as to the ways and means of evaluating and addressing the provision of care, the needs of the patients, the philosophy and operational policy to ensure that the day care centre continues to develop to meet the changing needs of the patients in the community.

Quizzes

Quizzes presented to a group in a sensitive and non-threatening manner can be an excellent means of facilitating communication amongst patients.

Prepared quizzes, tapes and books can often prove to be an expensive medium. However, with a little thought and imagination, staff can produce their own material that is ultimately appropriate to their patient group.

The following is a list of suggestions to be interpreted at a local level:

- Local history
- Sports
- Gardening
- Cookery
- Newspapers
- Music
- Everyday sounds/objects
- Tactile and taste
- TV and films
- Numbers
- Themes – countries, e.g. Italy, France, Australia

See also Communication and Group dynamics.

Reality of orientation

Keeping in touch with the real world may be achieved through a variety of means. For many elderly people, days and weeks roll into one: in-patients certainly lose touch with days of the week.

A wipe board with the day's date situated in day care and a stimulating notice board, changing every month, may give visual impact and link events of that month and/or events celebrated in the calendar. Newspaper quizzes or discussion groups can focus on the here and now of recent events and help patients keep in touch.

Referral criteria

Referral criteria should be included in the operational policy.

Relaxation

The ultimate benefit of relaxation is for patients to recognise their own stresses, anxieties and situations that induce such feelings and thus develop coping mechanisms and techniques to manage them.

Relaxation should be taught individually or to small groups building on existing techniques. Those who teach relaxation must have a positive belief towards its use themselves.

Reminiscence

To facilitate reminiscence and group discussion, quizzes, object recognition, auditory stimulation, slide shows, videos and significant events can all be used. This is useful for patients with recent memory loss as it enables them to contribute to the activity of the day.

Review of day care patients

Patients should regularly be reviewed with regard to their attendance in day care by members of the multi-disciplinary team involved in their care, justifying that their needs are still being addressed and cannot be met by another local service.

The issue of long-term attendees to many day care centres continues to be an ongoing management problem. One must question the ultimate benefit to such patients who have observed so many others come and go and, by process of elimination, await their turn.

Sensitive management is necessary with regard to patients whose symptoms or reason for referral have stabilised. This may result in a reduction of their days of attendance, movement to another day center locally or to a luncheon club. All have to be considered, ensuring that contact is maintained with an open door re-referral should the situation change.

As a cautionary note, it is an unhealthy environment where staff have favourites or develop a dependency upon their patients.

Salt dough

The use of salt dough is a cheap activity with a readily available material source. It can be used in a variety of ways, shapes and forms, and is ideal for group projects, such as Christmas decorations, or individual projects, such as picture frames, bowls or wall plaques. It can be enjoyed by both males and females, with patients easily becoming engrossed.

Basic recipe:
   3 cups of plain flour
   1 cup of salt
   Drizzle of oil
   Water to bind the dough mixture

Knead until smooth. Place in a plastic bag to prevent mixture from drying out throughout use. Mould into shape and bake at a low temperature until fully cooked and dried out (a hollow sound when tapped indicates that it is ready).

If a hook is required for the end product to hang on the wall this must be included prior to cooking the dough (paper clips, snapped in half, can be very useful). Baked dough can be varnished, painted or both for a finished end result.

When initially using salt dough it may be more successful if the group completes the activity together, stage by stage.

Speakers/slide shows

Outside speakers do provide an added interest to day care, often facilitating discussion amongst patients. However, it is important to ensure that the length of the talk is appropriate to patients' concentration span. Approximately 30 minutes is probably enough, as a warm environment and lights turned down (for a slide show) encourage patients to snooze. It is, therefore, useful to establish some form of communication with the presenter to help them recognise the patients' threshold and whether the talk needs to be cut short.

Subjects that may be well received are those of common interest to all. Local libraries may hold lists of contacts who will give talks, many of which are free, e.g. travel, local history, nature and wildlife.

Theme days

Theme days are particularly useful following the 'low' period after Christmas. An idea could be to select a country as the theme for the whole day, with day care decorated with flags, bunting, pictures, posters and colours of the country's flag. The morning session could be based on a quiz including general information relating to that country, e.g. a crossword, anagrams of towns or famous places, or patients guess or mark where historic/tourist sites are on a map.

The lunch table could be laid with napkins, etc., in the colours of the flag. The meal could have an element of the cuisine of the country with appropriate background music.

The afternoon activity, with some thought, could make a tentative link to the country, with material collected from tourist boards, embassies or travel agents.

As an example, an Italian theme day could run as follows:

- A quiz during the morning session based on general knowledge of Italy, such as famous sites, food, sports, cars, guessing the location of towns on a map and surrounding countries.
- A lunch of minestrone soup, lasagne, green salad and garlic bread, followed by Italian ice creams or tiramisu pudding.
- A pottery group during the afternoon session creating a ceramic tile each of which could eventually form a display.

Patients could dress appropriately.

Transport

Transport provision for day care has to be interpreted at local level, the main influence being that of the catchment area of the service and financial implications. However, the service must be appropriate to the needs of the patients.

Bussing patients to day care often has associations with ambulance transport rounds to hospital appointments and adds considerable duration to the patient's day.

For those centres utilising volunteer drivers, the usual selection criteria by voluntary service coordinators should be in place. Drivers must undertake lifting and handling training annually, and budget must be included in the overall day care financial management for the mileage allowances paid to volunteers.

Inevitably some patients, for example full time wheelchair users, will need access to ambulance transport.

Videos

Videos should not be seen as an easy means of occupying a patient group. If they are to be used patients should select their choice of viewing, going with the decision of the majority. Staff should give great consideration to the length of the video with respect to concentration spans and patient fatigue.

Should a video session be included in the activity programme for a social/entertainment purpose, then the addition of choc ices and microwave popcorn can enhance the event.

Videos can be used as a resource for reminiscence, such as video tapes solely depicting the events of a specific year. These do require pre-watching and editing by staff, as viewing the whole tape can become tedious.

Videos can be used to facilitate an introduction to other groups, e.g. watching the making of a Christmas cake, à la Delia Smith,[9] before the group attempts the activity for themselves.

Volunteers

It is important that careful selection criteria be implemented with regard to volunteer drivers and those spending time in day care. Volunteers in day care often have the closest patient contact within the centre.

A job description can identify clear roles and be a useful tool should problems arise. New volunteers should have a probationary period, and they must attend lifting and handling sessions and fire lectures regularly.

If day care centres recognise the value and contribution of volunteers, and are committed to the development of the service, then they should encourage their volunteers to undergo annual appraisals.

Woodwork

Woodwork projects can be bought in pre-cut, ready-to-assemble packs from a variety of craft suppliers. A point to note is the difference in wood quality, cut shapes, rough edges, inclusion of glue and nails, etc.

Large woodwork projects should not be undertaken as they take a great amount of space, storage and time to complete, many patients not seeing the end result. Woodwork should not take over the day centre, but it should be one of many activities included in the programme.

Hammers and small tools should be purchased: donated second-hand tools may be unsafe to use. Wooden headed hammers make less noise. Even so, patients with hearing aids could find woodwork sessions difficult to tolerate.

Varnishes, paint, glue and white spirit should be stored in a fire retardant, lockable cupboard away from direct patient access. Owing to COSHH Regulations[10] a list must be kept of the contents of the cupboard and the health and safety representative informed.

Writing, creative writing, story telling

Some patients may initially find this activity threatening, but if presented to a group of patients appropriately the response can be amazing.

Should such an activity be introduced to day care, it is beneficial to start with 'safe' subjects, to focus on happy events, remembering to end the group with positive feedback. As skills develop, or there is an acceptance of writing, more difficult topics can be approached, such as those including thoughts, feelings and emotions and sensitive memories.

In a group situation one would present the subject/topic, then ask patients to think for a set length of time about it, writing down comments or descriptions of the subject. It may then be possible for patients to share with the group, in turn, what they have written.

This can also be useful for those centres with in-patients. On a one-to-one basis, comments and writings are often insightful means of expression and communication, and can be of immense benefit to loved ones, often expressing things that were left unsaid.

Year book

The year book can take the form of a photograph album or scrap book, and could include a record of the year's events, photographs and creative writings, etc. This can be useful for patients who wish to reflect and remember other members of the group, but it can be equally beneficial with new members to 'get the feel' of what goes on.

A year book can also be a useful means of explaining the service provision to professional visitors.

Yearly programme

Time should be taken in putting together a well-structured programme of activities. Careful consideration should be given to events within the calendar year that could provide a focus, with especial planning around the low times to provide a boost, e.g. the gloom of winter, the low after Christmas.

The activity programme should be an equal responsibility of all members of the day care team, with time allocated to individual staff for preparation of group activities.

For those centres with in-patients who may attend day care, activities should not be repeated throughout a patient's stay. Care should be taken in the planning to consider this.

Activity should not be used as a diversion. It should be well planned and well structured in order to ensure that the patient achieves maximum satisfaction, success and confidence.

Yes

If a patient asks for something it should be achievable (if it is realistic). Day care cannot facilitate trips to the moon, but it should be recognised that it is worth asking!!

ZZZZZZZ!

Day care should not have the image of 'sit and knit' nor 'granny-sitting service' providing respite for carers.

Patients should return home after a stimulating day tired and in need of sleep. It should not be a place where people doze from boredom.

Conclusion

The conclusion I leave to the patients:

'At first I didn't want to come to day care. I must have been one of the most difficult people to try and persuade to give it a try! Eventually I decided to try it for myself and it's one of the best decisions I have ever made. There are lots of things going on – different activities to suit everyone's taste. Everyone is very kind and helpful – nothing's too much trouble. I would say to anyone – give it a try!'

'When day care was mentioned to me I did not like the idea because I am active and I didn't want to sit around moping. My welfare officer suggested the hospice and on my first day I was greeted at the door. I came in and immediately felt at home.'

'I couldn't have asked for a better welcome. I find it hard to describe, but you couldn't be unhappy here.'

'I enjoy the different activities and I have even had a go at painting! I also enjoy my meals and a can of mild! It makes my hair curl!'

Patient extracts from Creating Writing Group (1994)

References

1. The Food Hygiene (General) Regulations 1970 [SI 1970 No 1172] (ISBN 0-11-001172-4).
2. British Register of Complementary Practitioners – Institute of Complementary Medicine, PO Box 194, London, SE16 1QZ.
3. Food Safety Act 1990 (ISBN 0-10-541690-8).
4. Guidance on Manual Handling of Loads in the Health Services, Health Services Advisory Committee (ISBN 0-110886354-1).
5. Food Safety Act 1990 (ISBN 0-10-541690-8).
6. The Food Hygiene (General) Regulations 1970 [SI 1970 No. 1172] (ISBN 0-11-001172-4).
7. Willson M. *Occupational therapy in long-term psychiatry*. London: Churchill Livingstone, 1983.
8. Maslow AH. *The farther reaches of human nature*. Harmondsworth: Penguin, 1973.
9. Smith D. *Delia Smith's Christmas*. BBC Publications, 1991.
10. Control of Substances Hazardous to Health Regulations, 1988 (ISBN 0-11-8855336).

Further reading

Alen-Buckley C. *Sounds nostalgic, radio theme tunes from the 40s and 50s*. Bicester: Winslow Press, 1992.

Alen-Buckley C. *Sounds nostalgic, voices from the 40s and 50s*. Bicester: Winslow Press, 1991.

Campbell J. *Creative art in groupwork*. Bicester: Winslow Press, 1993.

Dynes R. *Creative writing in groupwork*. Bicester: Winslow Press, 1988.

Hagedorn R. *Therapeutic horticulture*. Nottingham: Nottingham Rehab, 1991.

Johnson PD. *Clay modelling for everyone*. Tunbridge Wells: Search Press, 1988.

Jones T. *Musical quiz*. Bicester: Winslow Press, 1988.

Liebmann M. *Art therapy for groups*. London: Routledge, 1991.
Organ, S. *How to make salt dough models*. Tunbridge Wells: Search Press, 1993.
Sherman, M. *The reminiscence quiz book*. Bicester: Winslow Press, 1991.

Useful addresses

Association of Professional Music Therapists, St Lawrence's Hospital, Caterham, Surrey.

BACUP, (Diet and the Cancer Patient, 1992). 3, Bath Place, Rivington Street, London, EC2A 3JR.

The Body Shop International plc, West Sussex, BN17 6LS.

British Association of Art Therapists, c/o 13c Northwood Road, London, N6.

British Red Cross Society, 9 Grosvenor Crescent, London, SW1X 7EJ.

British Society for Music Therapy, 69 Avondale Avenue, East Barnet, Hertfordshire, EN4 8NB.

The Council for Music in Hospitals, 74 Queens Road, Hersham, Surrey, ICT12 SLW.

Hospice Arts, Forbes House, 9 Artillery Lane, London, E1 7LP.

The Institute of Complementary Medicine, PO Box 194, London, SE16 1QZ.

International Federation of Aromatherapists, Stamford House, 2/4 Chiswick High Road, London, W4 1TH (Send £2 and A5 SAE for list of courses).

National Listening Library, 12 Lant Street, London, SE1 1QH.

Pets as Therapy, PRO Dogs, Rocky Bank, 4 New Road, Ditton, Maidstone, Kent, ME20 6AD.

RNIB Talking Book Service, Mount Pleasant, Wembley, Middlesex, HA10 1RR.

21

Social work in the palliative day care setting

Gillian Luff

Social work plays an integral part in the overall aims and strategy of the palliative day care team, which works towards achieving the dignity, independence and well-being of day care centre patients and their carers.

Where the social worker is a fully integrated team member a positive model of work may develop which allows for both continuity and flexibility of approach. Sensitive and appropriate support can be offered, from early diagnosis of illness through to help in bereavement if required.

Three major areas require careful thought when setting up the role of social worker and developing it appropriately in the day care setting:

- First, there needs to be a clear understanding of the specialist skills and knowledge he/she will be able to bring to the multi-disciplinary team, which will directly benefit patients, their carers, families and friends.
- Second, it should be recognised that the social worker brings important values and reflects key issues in society. These include the commitment to equality of access and opportunity to all groups in society and the demonstration of respect for other people's individuality. There will be a positive role to play in helping the day centre aim for and establish good anti-discriminatory and anti-racist practice.
- Thirdly, the management and the funding of the post with its back-up services and resources should be clearly defined along with lines of responsibility and support.

Specialist skills

Traditionally in the health care field, the social work role may be identified with welfare rights issues, pensions, grants, housing, nursing home applications and packages of care, etc. As Maslow identified in his description of a hierarchy of needs,[1] food and shelter issues may be paramount and must indeed be addressed, but in the complicated area of palliative care, these major issues will be vying with other equally pressing ones, such as loss of independence, anxieties about the family or friends, fears about the future, both short-term and long-term, body image, sexuality, the unknown, etc. The patient or the carer may indeed begin by testing out the social worker, presenting safer practical issues before moving on to the more complex social and personal areas of concern.

The specialist skills which the social worker brings will enable him/her to make a thorough assessment of the person/family in the situation, taking account of

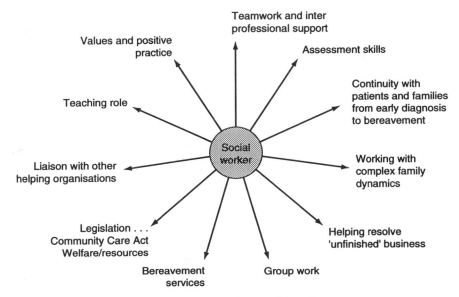

Fig. 21.1 The role of the social worker.

wider, holistic issues. By working with the whole family and carer network it will be possible to develop a plan which recognises the important practical needs and seeks ways of helping the user remedy these, whilst establishing a flexible plan for good, psychosocial support appropriate to the current situation.

The social worker will be using cognitive and interpersonal skills to evaluate and clarify the situation and to make and sustain good working relationships.[2] The social worker will also be reflecting on and trying to understand the strong feelings and emotions which emerge both in themselves and in the patients and their carers, as issues of loss, sadness, anger, guilt or relief rise to the surface.

Recognising these complex feelings, the social worker will be well aware of his/her own need for support or consultation on a regular basis, which can be so constructive in avoiding the pitfall of 'burnout' for professional carers. Self awareness remains a key developmental issue. Within the multi–disciplinary team in the day care setting there will be opportunities for informal mutual support. The social worker may, however, be instrumental in setting up a more formal approach to staff support by canvassing for and establishing whether colleagues would value this. An external consultant may be chosen to fulfil this role, who will offer a confidential forum for discussion, without reporting back in detail to the management team.

The support needs of volunteers can be overlooked too and the social worker, in conjunction with other team members, may offer structured support to these important carers, whose strong sense of idealism may make them particularly vulnerable to stress and burnout.

Group or individual support, usually led by the social worker, will be a major requirement for volunteers who take part in the work of the bereavement service, both to ensure the maintenance of a high standard of service and to provide essential ongoing learning opportunities. This vital support cannot be neglected. It reduces the tendency for volunteers to carry an unnecessarily heavy emotional load.

The whole subject area of group work is one in which most social workers have developed important skills. The day centre setting offers an appropriate opportunity for using these skills and for working closely with other members of the multi-disciplinary team to facilitate user groups.[3]

Day patients are by definition well enough to make the necessary effort to attend their day centre setting. Whilst there, they may be able to tolerate and make use of a safe, gently structured, well-negotiated group in which the members, rather than the facilitators, set the agenda and establish group rules, side-stepping some of the more traditional group norms to take account of emotional needs, physical frailty, etc.

The group may work well in these circumstances if allowed to be self selecting and tolerant of less than regular attendance. Minimal interpretation of events and feelings may be required of the facilitators whose task is mainly that of providing basic safety rules and maintaining appropriate time limits for the group.

The group members may challenge the medical model and the helping professionals' cherished beliefs. This needs to be heard and acknowledged. They will probably wish to vent their frustrations and irritations and to express how it feels to be stigmatised as a result of having a diagnosis of terminal illness. None the less, while they control the choice and level of subject matter, a lively atmosphere of exchange and support may emerge along with a strong sense of companionship in which group members retain their dignity, power and independence.

Without doubt, the National Health Service and Community Care Act 1990 has heralded important and complex changes to the role of the social worker. Other significant legislation which has a bearing on social work in the day care setting is the Children Act 1989 and the Chronically Sick and Disabled Persons Act 1970. The major impact, however, is that of the community care legislation which has been felt most keenly at hospice in-patient unit level but has also strongly influenced the way in which the day care social worker must interact and negotiate on behalf of user groups. Social Service departments, formerly the providers of services, must now handle the complexities of both purchasing and sometimes providing, services linking public and private provision. The social worker will need to negotiate skilfully with the Social Services department, voluntary or private agencies, primary health care teams and health services such as hospitals. This has generated an increase in work for all concerned.

The intentions of the White Paper, *Caring for people*, 1989[4] were entirely laudable:

> Community care means providing the services and support which people who are affected by problems of ageing, mental illness, mental handicap or physical or sensory disability, need to be able to live as independently as possible in their own homes or in homely settings in the community.

The report went on to recognise that community care should be flexible and sensitive to the needs of individuals and their carers, allowing for a large range of options, while none the less concentrating on those with greatest need. Choice and independence for service users were to be the cornerstones of the policy.

The social worker's role in assessment of need, designing appropriate 'packages of care', purchasing and arranging delivery of these services, has varied according to employment status with Social Services departments. Independently funded social workers, employed directly by their day care organisation, may be dependent on a complex and sometimes cumbersome system of case allocation and assessment of need by the local Social Services department. Where this role of assessment is carried out by the specialist day care social worker, they will, however, be acutely sensitive to a sick or weary patient's needs and will recognise that the process of assessment and appropriate communication with the patient will need to be very flexible. Ten or fifteen minutes can be a very long period for an unwell or weak person to concentrate on such tasks and this must be respected.

A wide geographic spread of service users may entail complex negotiations with different budgetary authorities. To complicate matters further, the internal market within the Health Services has generally led to a reduction in beds available for some groups of elderly and infirm patients, who may now need to be accommodated in private nursing homes with heavy cost implications for the local authority community care budget. This may in turn diminish the options available for patients as risk assessment categories are tightened and may reduce the length of time that day care patients can maintain dignity and independence in their own homes. The social worker's role is that of advocate, fighting for the patients' right to maintain an independent status for as long as they and their carers wish.

The role of advocate extends to that of welfare rights. Social workers involved in the palliative care movement have led important campaigns to help individuals and families obtain appropriate financial support, such as the Attendance Allowance, without having to prove need for a waiting period of 6 months. The focus is now shifting to widowers, treated unequally in Britain at present in terms of financial support following a partner's death. Examples of hardship caused by the present unequal situation help to promote a strong case for change in the law.

The multi-disciplinary team may be acutely aware of complex and difficult, stormy or resentful dynamics within partnerships, exacerbated by illness and impending loss. Social workers are well versed in the task of dealing with difficult dynamics. By using their understanding of family systems theory and drawing on counselling skills and much sensitivity, they may be able to move partners or family members forward to the point where they can address some of the major unfinished business, thus working towards the core issues of saying 'I'm sorry', 'Thank you' and 'I love you', which can have such a significant effect upon the ability to cope later with bereavement.

For example, a woman had divorced her exasperating husband, who had spent most of his adult life fearing he had a cancer. He had watched his own mother die in difficult and painful circumstances while he was a young adolescent and had a great dread of illness, thus magnifying every common ache and pain. Three months after the divorce, he was diagnosed with cancer, already too malignant to be cured. His ex-wife promptly remarried him and became very over-protective towards him, in relation to the palliative care support services. Anger and guilt were strong emotions shown by both partners – they spent some very volatile and chaotic times back together, complicated by the pressure of adolescent teenagers.

The husband attended the day centre on a weekly basis, which offered a much-needed break for all the family. The social worker worked closely with the other team members, seeing the husband regularly at the day centre. The wife was seen at home, separately. The work moved on to important family discussions which drew in the teenagers who were feeling extremely marginalised and ill informed.

They all completed most of the tasks of dealing with their unfinished business and were able to say appropriate, if very emotional, goodbyes. Support was needed for a while in bereavement, but the process did not become unduly complicated.

Members of the multi-disciplinary team are often called upon to teach about palliative care – social workers are no exception. It is an important and vital part of the original vision of Dame Cicely Saunders which social workers within the hospice movement have embraced more readily than that of writing or research. Health care professionals, clergy, teachers and voluntary groups have readily joined in active social work teaching sessions built around an understanding of loss and change, family dynamics, communication skills, ethical issues, etc.

The provision of a bereavement service has been an essential part of palliative care from the earliest days. Where day centres are a part of a hospice centre, they may well have direct access to the existing bereavement service. Social workers have been involved from the outset with selecting, training, supporting and developing this work using carefully chosen volunteers who contribute a great deal to the provision of an effective service.[5]

Many families can and do cope within their own support structures as they go through the process of bereavement. But where individuals and families find themselves struggling deeply and feel unsupported, the bereavement team will provide structured planned support to enable people to work through Worden's four stages of grief,[6] building upon the family's or individual's own coping strength.

The social worker is likely to be involved in some of the more complex bereavements where chronic or complicated grief is a feature or where grieving children and adolescents present important needs. Occasionally, the risk of suicide becomes apparent and the social worker will work closely with the primary health care team and psychiatric services to ensure the grieving person gets the appropriate support. Social work skills will be called upon where a history of earlier child abuse severely complicates a later dependent relationship. For instance, a daughter who finds herself in the caring role for her father, who had subjected her to abuse as a child or adolescent, experiences a wide range of conflicting and painful emotions. These complex feelings may not be revealed until the father dies, at which point the carer may begin to deal with her own loss of childhood and adolescence as well as her strong emotions towards her dead father.

An overview of some of the key areas of possible social work involvement may be shown in diagrammatic form and by case illustration (Figure 21.2).

A terminally ill young mother may have the deepest anxieties for her primary school aged children. She may worry about her partner's ability to cope with her care and about the setting up of a suitable plan for their family's short- and long-term future. The mother may have many anxieties about how and when to tell the children of her impending death and how to maintain a healthy ongoing environment in the intervening months or years before she dies.

If there are additional worries, such as reduced income because she has ceased work, or if her partner's job is threatened, due to caring responsibilities, the burden of overload and anxiety will be immense. The social worker may be able to ensure she applies for financial support via the Disabled Living Allowance, or negotiates suitable financial support from her employer. The social worker may encourage the young mother to prepare the children's school staff and may also

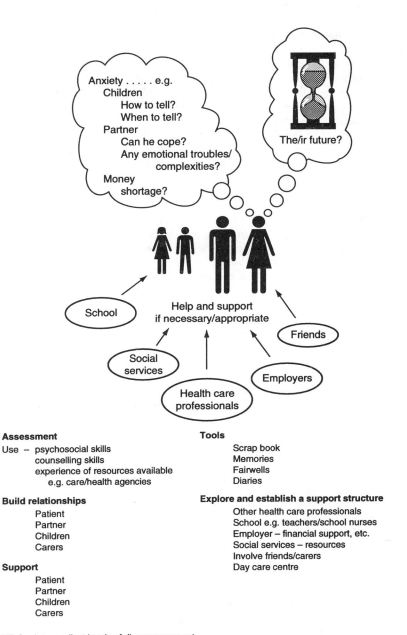

Anxiety . . . . . e.g.
Children
How to tell?
When to tell?
Partner
Can he cope?
Any emotional troubles/
complexities?
Money
shortage?

The/ir future?

School

Help and support
if necessary/appropriate

Social
services

Friends

Health care
professionals

Employers

Assessment

Use – psychosocial skills
counselling skills
experience of resources available
e.g. care/health agencies

Build relationships

Patient
Partner
Children
Carers

Support

Patient
Partner
Children
Carers

Tools

Scrap book
Memories
Fairwells
Diaries

Explore and establish a support structure

Other health care professionals
School e.g. teachers/school nurses
Employer – financial support, etc.
Social services – resources
Involve friends/carers
Day care centre

NB Seek to readjust levels of disempowerment

Fig. 21.2 Example – the terminally ill young mother.

offer guidance and support to the front line teachers if they have little experience or skill in dealing with such life-shattering events. If the family gives consent, liaison with other health care professionals, such as health visitors and GPs, may be appropriate.

Four or five well-planned sessions with the mother, or both partners at this early stage, at home or in the day care centre or a mix of both, may give the partners the necessary confidence to develop a workable plan for managing the children's and their own emotional needs. Good communication and close liaison will be essential in this process which will probably be multi-disciplinary, involving shared work with the day centre team or domiciliary nurses. The work might involve creating journals, books of memories, building up support structures of friends, services, etc., 'hoping for the best', whilst 'preparing for the worst'.

As the illness progresses and greater dependency needs are identified, the social worker may become more actively involved, building on the earlier good relationship, greatly encouraging the family to tackle problems openly and honestly. There may be a need for increased support from the community social services and a plan may be made for the early stages of bereavement to ensure safety and continuity for the children. The social worker may continue to support this family to a lesser or greater degree during quite a lengthy period in bereavement. The major role may be that of working with the father, rather than directly with the children but by this point, however, there is a strong chance that the social worker will be well known to the children and well accepted. This is a model for future mental health rather than mental disease, building on people's ability to cope and manage their grief.

Values and anti-discriminatory practice

Social workers will have a commitment to a set of values which involve concepts such as social justice and social welfare, enhancing the life of individuals, families and groups and the repudiation of all forms of negative discrimination.[7] They will share many of these values with other team members; for instance respect for the dignity of individuals, the right to maintain privacy and confidentiality and for patients and families to choose their own preferred outcomes, wherever possible. Sheldon[8] reminds us of the further underpinning values which professionals need when communicating successfully with patients and carers. These include a non-judgemental approach, respect for the uniqueness of each individual and the ability to offer an empathetic response. Further qualities involve genuineness, self awareness and a 'positive belief in the potential of individuals for change, even when they face the crisis of death'.[9]

Having a terminal illness such as AIDS or cancer can be a paralysing and isolating experience as a result of the attitude of others, which may actively or passively stigmatise and disempower both patients and their carers. The social worker can play an important role in partnership with the ill or disabled person, to reduce the emphasis upon the medical model of illness and to focus instead upon maximising an individual's potential.[10] The day centre setting provides the opportunity to reduce negative attitudes, encourages patients to revalue themselves, take initiatives once more and control their own lives. But it is still rare for a patient or carer to be included upon management committees, where they could give appropriate feedback on the services provided.

In Britain, the majority of hospices have been established within leafy, spacious middle-class districts. User groups do not reflect the multi-cultural nature of our society or the full spread of social classes. This raises a number of questions which social workers and researchers may wish to probe. Do referring agencies make assumptions about which groups in society will want to use such facilities? What can be done to ascertain the extent of need and to make the provision of services accessible to all regardless of ethnic origin, culture, religion, background, gender and beliefs? Separate works by Rees,[11] and O'Neill[12] in recent years, have drawn attention to the discrepancy between the provision of palliative care services and their take-up by different ethnic and religious groups in our society. Oliviere[13] reminds us that a service will only be available to all if it is set up 'to give the appropriate message that all groups are welcome and if we as individuals are as comfortable as possible in working with people of differing cultural experiences and backgrounds'. For instance, one way of creating a more accessible and welcoming day centre unit is by making positive arrangements for different diets and food preparation; also for differing religious customs.

Social work skills will be called upon to help assess which aspects of the patient's cultural background are important to them in the face of terminal illness. They may draw in resources such as interpreters and arrange for the translation of literature into local languages. The social worker can work with other team members to make personal contact with local leaders or to provide day care open days; support can be gained for tackling the image of the service and in targeting the sources of referrals such as local general practitioners, with the aim of making the service accessible to all who may need it.

Where the day centre setting is a free-standing facility or the 'parent' hospice provides more than one day centre location, there is the clear opportunity to serve a broader mix of society, which should be seized. Added to this, where staff and volunteers reflect a multi-cultural diverse society, there is a strong chance that the service will be responsive and acceptable to people of differing backgrounds. By emphasising the adaptive qualities of the service, meeting the various needs of different cultures, we can move away from the model of making the patient fit the service as provided.

The hospice movement has led the way in so much that has been positive for the person or family facing terminal illness and should continue to be at the forefront in reviewing and developing services which are accessible to all who need them, regardless of ethnic origin, culture, gender, creed or belief. The day centre which addresses these issues may begin by establishing an equal opportunities policy for staff patients and carers. An accepted policy of education and training, which is embraced by the management as well as staff and volunteers, is an important first step in that direction.

Management and funding of the post

Day centres vary considerably in their funding and management structure and whether they are attached to or separate from a local hospice unit. Their general ethos will also probably vary according to how closely they are associated with such a unit. These factors will have an impact upon the financing and organisation of the social work post.

The case has already been stated for the social worker to be a fully integrated member of the day centre team. However, a plea should be made from the outset for consultation with well-established palliative care social workers, possibly through the auspices of their professional association, who could offer helpful guidelines and support in the early development of such posts. Where the post is a 'core position' it is important to investigate and establish lines of support which will be available to the social worker. The funding of the post has implications for both the management and the lines of responsibility.

There are three major options:

1. Funding by voluntary sources, local or national.
2. Funding by local authority Social Services department.
3. A mix of both 1 and 2.

Each choice has its advantages and disadvantages (Figure 21.3).

Lines of responsibility remain a thorny issue to clarify and are subject to much discussion. Ideally, the social worker shares a management role with the nursing and medical professionals within this small multi-disciplinary team. In practice in free-standing day centres, or larger centres attached to hospice units, a manager is designated and is often from a nursing or medical background.

Whichever situation prevails, it will be important to establish clear lines of communication and a well-defined role. However, flexibility should not be sacrificed and the post holder should be able to develop interests which fit the overall aims and objectives of the day centre. The social worker will sometimes be accountable to a manager within the 'umbrella' hospice organisation. This person may be a social work team leader or a medical/nursing manager. Alternatively, the social worker may report direct to the Social Services manager.

The post of social worker in the day care setting requires certain very positive attributes, well-established social work expertise, coupled with a good team work approach, communications skills and the ability to stand on one's own feet. Furthermore, the post holder will require personal maturity and the ability to manage the post resourcefully.

	Advantage	Disadvantage
Voluntary sector post, locally or nationally funded	☺ Autonomy ☺ Less bureaucracy ☺ Full attention given to aims of the day centre	☹ Funds may be low ☹ Full-time post may not be possible
Local Authority Social Service funding	☺ Faster access to resources/careplans ☺ Part of a large social work team	☹ Bureaucratic ☹ Cutbacks may occur ☹ Day centre may cross several area boundaries
Part funded on a voluntary sector basis, part funded by Local Authority	☺ A foot in both camps! ☺ Access to resources	☹ 'Scapegoating' ☹ Difficult to define clear procedures or lines of responsibility

Fig. 21.3 Advantages and disadvantages of the funding types.

Lastly, the post should be properly resourced with adequate working accommodation, access to private interview space, secretarial/clerical support, travelling allowance and telephones. It is worth remembering here that resources should include access to books, support and further training to refresh and renew dedicated staff whose batteries must be recharged if they are to continue the process of working intensively with dying patients and their carers and families.

In conclusion, the social worker has a valuable contribution to make to the fully effective day centre setting, bringing skills, knowledge and values which will complement those of other team members. The social worker will have in mind the need to create a positive and welcoming environment for all who require the service and will particularly emphasise its 'emotional accessibility'. The aim will be to create a service which is equitable, accessible and acceptable to all.

References

1. Maslow AH. *Motivation and personality*. New York: Harper and Row, 1954.
2. CCETSW, (Central Council for Education and Training in Social Work) *Rules and requirements for the diploma in social work*, Paper 30, 2nd edn. London: CCETSW, 1991.
3. Carter P. *The Thursday Group*. Hospice Bulletin, Issue No. 24, The Hospice Information Service at St Christopher's Hospice, October 1994.
4. Department of Health, White Paper, Cmd 849, *Caring for people: community care in the next decade and beyond*. London: HMSO, 1989.
5. Earnshaw-Smith E, Yorkstone P. *Setting up and running a bereavement service*. St Christopher's Hospice, 1986.
6. Worden JW. *Grief counselling and grief therapy*, 2nd edn. London: Routledge, 1991.
7. CCETSW (Central Council for Education and Training in Social Work) *Rules and requirements for the Diploma in Social Work*, Paper 30, Section 2.2. London, CCETSW, 1991.
8. Sheldon F. Communication In: Saunders C, Sykes N, eds *The management of terminal malignant disease*, 3rd edn. London: Edward Arnold, 1993.
9. Ibid.
10. Thompson N. *Anti-discriminatory practice*. London: Macmillan, 1993.
11. Rees D. Immigrants and the hospice: *Health Trends* 1986; **18**: 89–91.
12. O'Neill JM. Ethnic minorities – neglected by palliative care providers: *J Cancer Care* 1994; **3**(4): 215–20.
13. Oliviere D. Cross-cultural principles of care. In: Saunders C, Sykes N, eds *The management of terminal malignant disease*, 3rd edn. London: Edward Arnold, 1993; 203.

Further reading

Firth S. Cultural issues in terminal care. In: Clark D, ed. *The future of palliative care*. London: Open University Press, 1993.

Green J. *Death with dignity*, Vols 1 and 2. Nursing Times Publications, 1991.

Monroe B. Social work in palliative care. In: Doyle D, Hanks G, Macdonald N, eds *Oxford textbook of palliative medicine*. Oxford: Oxford University Press, 1993; 565–74.

Neuberger J. *Caring for dying people of different faiths*, 2nd edn. London: Wolfe, 1994.

22

Lymphoedema clinic

Caroline Badger

Introduction

Any attempt to provide a palliative care service to patients with advanced disease should give serious consideration to the problem of oedema. There are many types of oedema, of which lymphoedema is just one form. Cancer is probably the major cause of lymphoedema in Britain[1] and while reliable figures on the incidence of lymphoedema among cancer patients (other than breast cancer patients) are rare, clinical experience suggests that it is a significant problem.

Other forms of oedema, such as that resulting from dependency or immobility of limbs, or hypoproteinaemia, are commonly seen among elderly, debilitated, paralysed or immobile patients and are therefore to be expected in a palliative care setting.[2] The word lymphoedema is used here for simplicity but it acknowledges that many of the oedemas seen in palliative care are of a mixed origin and often involve the venous as well as the lymphatic system.

The decision to develop a lymphoedema clinic within a palliative day care unit must take into account the needs of the population that it serves: different groups of patients will have different needs at different stages of their condition. The extent and nature of services that can be provided are reviewed here together with a brief outline of the different services each will require.

Approaches to the management of oedema can largely be divided into three main types:

1. intensive treatment;
2. palliative treatment;
3. maintenance and monitoring.

Each of these approaches requires different resources and each has different implications in terms of the time and level of expertise needed to deliver care.

Intensive treatment

Treatment skills

Intensive treatment (or 'complex decongestive therapy' as it is known throughout the rest of Europe) is the term used to describe a course of treatment given to the patient by a suitably skilled therapist (be it nurse or physiotherapist) with the aim of reducing the size of the limb, and restoring the shape and function of the limb to as close to the patient's normal as possible.

The treatment usually consists of:

* a daily programme of compression (at this stage often in the form of bandages);
* a specific form of massage known as manual lymph drainage;
* exercises to promote drainage and exercises to improve joint mobility;
* care of the skin.

A course of intensive treatment will last on average between 2 and 3 weeks.

Patients undergoing this type of treatment will usually be free of active cancer and have moderate to severe oedema.

The therapist delivering intensive treatment should be suitably experienced in all the various treatment techniques cited above, since clinical experience suggests that it is the combination of these different treatments that brings about the best results.

The skills required to perform this kind of treatment include:

* a comprehensive understanding of the anatomy and physiology of the lymphatic system;
* a thorough understanding of the mechanisms underlying the development of different types of oedema;
* the ability to make a thorough assessment of the patient's needs and to make a differential diagnosis between different types of oedema;
* an understanding of the aims and limitations of all the different modalities of treatment;
* the ability to apply external pressure safely and effectively, whether by use of multi-layer bandaging, compression hosiery or pneumatic compression;
* expertise in the treatment of the characteristic skin problems associated with chronic oedema;
* an understanding of the role of movement and positioning in the promotion of lymph drainage;
* the ability to perform manual lymph drainage;
* an understanding of, and proficiency in, the measurement of response to treatment;
* an understanding of the psychological and social implications for the patient, the family and the therapist of having to deal with a chronic and, as yet, incurable condition.

Suitable training for specialists is available ranging from training in the management of breast-cancer related lymphoedema of the upper limb, to the management of all types of chronic oedema.

Staff

Lymphoedema is an area of specialisation that attracts both physiotherapists and nurses. Regardless of which profession it is that is responsible for the intensive treatment, there is much to be gained from the involvement of both nurses and physiotherapists, since each brings particular areas of expertise relevant to the problem of oedema: for example skin hygiene and care are essential in order to combat the recurrent episodes of infection that are characteristic of lymphoedema, while joint mobility is almost always impaired in the lymphoedematous limb and restoration of a full range of movement has in turn a beneficial effect on the long-term control of oedema.

Whether part-time or full-time, the therapist must be sure to have a designated time each day for carrying out treatment. Treatment during this intensive phase is on a daily basis (weekends excluded) for several weeks at a time; unless there is designated time available the patient may get halfway through a course of intensive treatment only to find that other demands on the therapist's time mean that the course is cut short. Stopping and starting treatment, even if for short periods, will almost certainly reduce its effectiveness.

Patients benefit enormously from a multi-disciplinary approach to their care since oedema can result in a whole range of problems, restrictions and disabilities. Occupational therapists play an important role in allowing the patient to function as independently as possible. There is also a place for links with a dietician: obesity can stand in the way of a satisfactory response to treatment and appropriate dietary advice can ensure that treatment has the maximum effect possible.

As in any dealings with cancer patients, regular medical input is essential; recurrance or advancement of tumour must be recognised together with other medical conditions that might have an impact on oedema or its treatment.

Material resources

As well as designated treatment time there must be a designated area for assessment, treatment and follow-up. Whether a treatment area is shared or kept specifically for lymphoedema will depend on the size and frequency of the clinic and/or treatment sessions. An average treatment session for a single patient lasts about an hour; a longer appointment may be needed for an initial assessment of the patient's needs or if more than one limb is involved, conversely less time will be needed for a follow-up visit.

The facilities should include an adjustable height examination or massage couch and screens are essential to ensure privacy during examination and treatment. Patients undergoing bandaging should be able to wash the affected limb each day between changes of bandages.

There are a number of items that will need to be readily available if intensive treatment is to be offered. Multi-layer bandaging involves the use of several different materials including stockinette, sheets of soft foam, sheets of dense foam, soft wadding and short-stretch bandages. The amount of storage space required for these will depend on the numbers of patients treated but some storage space (preferably in the treatment area) will need to be provided. Stocks of off-the-shelf compression hosiery will again depend on the numbers of patients seen; different types of oedema and indeed different patients will require different classes of compression and different styles and sizes of hosiery; once again storage space will need to be allowed for.

Palliative treatment

Treatment skills

Palliative treatment is the term used to describe treatment aimed at relieving the symptoms associated with oedema rather than at reducing and controlling oedema long term. In cancer patients this is usually because a tumour is responsible for the oedema and unless the tumour can be influenced by treatment it is unlikely that control will be gained over the oedema.

The aims of this kind of treatment are therefore to identify what symptoms most distress the patient, be it a feeling of pressure in the limb, or stiff joints, or seepage of lymph from the skin (all common problems for these patients), and to try to alleviate them.

The techniques of treatment used in intensive treatment are adapted for use in relieving symptoms. Multi-layer bandaging, for example, may be used in palliative treatment but instead of compressing the limb in order to reduce the size the bandages are applied in such a way that they simply support the swollen tissues: the sensation of pressure within the limb is relieved without fluid being forced out of the limb through drainage routes which may be obstructed by tumour deposits.

Patients undergoing this type of treatment will usually have advanced cancer or arterial disease, and will often have widespread oedema involving large areas of the body as well as the limbs. They will typically have a short life expectancy.

The therapist delivering palliative care should be suitably experienced in the palliative application of the various treatment techniques already mentioned. In the palliative setting, treatment is not usually applied as a defined course but may be continued for as long as the effects are perceived to be beneficial. Treatments may be used on their own to achieve a particular and specific effect and need not necessarily be combined.

Ideally the skills required to perform this kind of treatment include:

- a thorough understanding of the mechanisms underlying the development of different types of oedema;
- the ability to make a thorough assessment of the patient's needs and to make a differential diagnosis between different types of oedema;
- an understanding of the aims and limitations of all the different modalities of treatment;
- the ability to apply support with either multi-layer bandaging or support hosiery;
- expertise in the treatment of the characteristic skin problems associated with advanced tumour;
- an understanding of the role of movement and positioning in the promotion of lymph drainage;
- the ability to perform simple lymph massage.

The need for education in palliative treatment is recognised and initiatives are underway to provide suitable training for those working in this field.

Staff

Providing palliation of the symptoms associated with oedema should be considered standard in any palliative day care unit, such as the ability to treat pain or nausea and vomiting are considered so now.

There is an argument for ensuring that all nurses and physiotherapists involved in palliative care have an understanding of the causes of oedema in advanced disease and have the skills to distinguish between the appropriateness of intensive treatment and the need for a palliative approach. The involvement of the rest of the multi-disciplinary team is as important in palliative treatment as in the intensive treatment phase. Dietary advice may be helpful in boosting hypo-proteinaemia; gentle exercises may preserve or increase joint mobility; aids may be available to compensate for reduced function in an oedematous limb. A close relationship with medical colleagues will ensure that drugs such as diuretics or steroids are used appropriately to reduce fluid overload or improve drainage, while those with fluid-retaining properties are kept to a minimum whenever possible.

Material resources

The material resources needed are much the same as for intensive treatment. The same bandage materials are needed for support bandaging as for compression bandaging. Generally speaking, the higher classes of compression hosiery are not required, Classes 1 and 2, in a range of sizes and styles, should meet the needs of most patients. Since hosiery typically has a useful life of around 6 months for stockings, or 3–4 months for arm sleeves, and their use in palliative treatment is often short term, many items can be recycled several times before they become redundant. Storage space, preferably close to the treatment area, will be required for all these items.

Maintenance and monitoring

Treatment skills

Maintenance treatment is the term used to describe treatment aimed at maintaining the degree of oedema and condition of the affected area. The kinds of patients requiring maintenance treatment are those whose oedema is insignificant, mild and uncomplicated (in which case they can bypass the intensive treatment and move straight to maintenance), or those who have had a successful course of intensive treatment (their oedema has been reduced and their condition improved and they now need to maintain the improvement).

Maintenance treatment is actually carried out by the patients themselves in their own homes, but before they can do this they need to be taught how to carry out a daily programme of care. Lymphoedema is a chronic, incurable condition and the patients will need to follow some sort of maintenance programme for the rest of their lives. The role of the health care professional in providing this kind of service is therefore twofold: teaching the patients how to manage their condition (gradually leading them towards an independent existence), and monitoring their condition long term, ready to step in if the condition worsens.

The programme of treatment used in maintenance treatment usually consists of compression hosiery, care of the skin, and exercise to improve drainage (with or without exercises to improve mobility or strength).

Monitoring consists of using a combination of objective measurements and subjective assessments to evaluate the response to treatment and to adapt the treatment programme to ensure the maximum desired effect. Should problems arise or the patient's condition worsen the health professional engaged in monitoring can ensure a prompt and appropriate referral to suitable members of the multi-disciplinary team.

Maintenance and monitoring represent the second stage of treatment for patients who have completed intensive treatment; whether provided separately by 'key workers' or provided by a lymphoedema specialist as an integral part of a lymphoedema service, maintenance and monitoring are crucial to the long-term control of oedema.

Ideally the skills required to provide this kind of care will include:

- an understanding of the anatomy and physiology of the lymphatic system;
- a thorough understanding of the mechanisms underlying the development of different types of oedema;
- an understanding of the aims and limitations of maintenance treatment;
- the ability to make an assessment of the patient's needs and to make appropriate referrals if the patient requires more than maintenance treatment.
- the ability to apply compression hosiery safely and effectively;
- expertise in the treatment of the characteristic skin problems associated with chronic oedema;
- an understanding of the role of movement and positioning in the promotion of lymph drainage;
- the ability to perform simple lymph massage;
- an understanding of, and proficiency in, the measurement of response to treatment;
- an understanding of the psychological and social implications for the patient, the family and the therapist of having to deal with a chronic and, as yet, incurable condition.
- the ability to teach the patient to care for themselves.

Multi-disciplinary educational courses are available for training in this level of care and these are often referred to as 'key worker' courses.

Staff

Maintenance and monitoring can be provided by a variety of different health care professionals (key workers) wherever patients at risk of developing, or having developed, oedema are to be found. It can, and probably should form part of the routine care of such patients.

Where intensive treatment is offered, maintenance and monitoring may be the responsibility of the lymphoedema specialist but a word of caution here. The long-term nature of any follow-up may mean that as more patients move from intensive to maintenance treatment the bulk of the specialist's time is spent on this second phase of care leaving less and less time for intensive treatment. The ideal situation would be to have key worker help with maintenance and monitoring (either attached to the clinic or outside in the community or out-patients of a local hospital, for example), leaving the specialist free to make more effective and efficient use of specialist skills.

Material resources

A designated treatment area (with an adjustable height couch) where regular out-patient clinics can be held is essential. A wide range of compression hosiery, in terms of compression classes, styles and sizes, will need to be kept in stock. Once again storage space, preferably close to the treatment area, will be required for all these items.

Lymphoedema clinic

The first step in planning a lymphoedema clinic should be to discover what kind of care is already being provided locally; this will help to ensure that any new service will enhance and complement existing care and will avoid unnecessary duplication.

Each of the approaches to treatment outlined above may be offered through an out-patient lymphoedema clinic. The extent to which the approaches are combined and offered through the same clinic will depend on the needs of the population that it serves and the availability of resources and treatment skills. If services are extended beyond 'in-house' patients it should be borne in mind that lymphoedema can affect non-cancer patients, and it is likely that once a clinic has become established referrals of non-cancer patients will almost certainly follow.

The range of skills, the philosophy of care and the tendency towards a relaxed, non-clinical environment make the palliative day care unit an ideal setting for a lymphoedema clinic.

References

1. Mortimer PS. Investigation and management of lymphoedema. *Vasc Med Rev*, 1990; 1: 1–20.
2. Badger C. Lymphoedema. In: Penson J, Fisher R, eds *Palliative care for people with cancer*, 2nd edn. London: Edward Arnold, 1995: 81–90.

Contacts regarding educational courses

Specialist course

Eunice Jeffs,
St Catherine's Hospice,
Malthouse Road,
Crawley, E. Sussex, RH10 6BH.

Palliative care course

Margaret Sneddon,
Macmillan Lecturer in Palliative Care,
Department of Postgraduate Medical Education,
University of Glasgow,
124 Observatory Road,
Glasgow G12 8UZ.

Key worker course

Jacqueline Todd,
Ardenlea Marie Curie Centre,
Ilkley, W. Yorkshire, LS29 9EM.

23

Complementary medicine

Sue Taylor

Fear knocked at the door –
Faith opened it.
There was no–one there ...

Old Chinese Proverb

Impact of a life-threatening illness engenders fear and uncertainty for patients and their families. Supportive therapies offered to people in this situation may enhance their ability to cope at this time. These services include a wide range of therapies which augment orthodox medicine and which may not be generally available in conventional treatment centres. There has been some controversy over what is meant by the terms used to describe these therapies. However, what's in a name? Quite a great deal, it would appear, as looking through some dictionary definitions revealed:[1]

- Alternative: two choices, replacing
- Unorthodox: incorrect, unsound
- Supplement: addition
- Diversional: turn aside, amuse
- Supportive: to bear, cherish
- Complementary: *something making up a whole.*

The complementary approaches which help to 'make up a whole' and which may be offered in palliative care include complementary therapies such as aromatherapy and reflexology, diversional therapies such as handicrafts, and stress-management techniques. An ideal setting for offering complementary therapies in palliative care as part of an holistic support service is in a community day care centre.

In his book *Supportive therapies in health care*, Wells (1994)[2] classifies complementary therapies as one aspect of a range of possible support for patients, which may be available alongside conventional treatment. However, according to Fisher and Ward a more accurate description of complementary therapies is that they are 'unconventional therapeutic methods'[3] because of the large number of therapies which are available outside orthodox treatment centres. Complementary therapies do attempt to move away from the traditional disease-orientated model and consequently, problems have arisen in integrating the two cultures: 'one driven by technology, the other by human need'.[4] However, in spite of the difficulties there has been a surge of interest in complementary therapies and in an attempt to respond to the perceived demand, consideration should be given in planning services to ensure that this support is offered. The setting where complementary therapies are offered should be a prime consideration. For many patients and their families returning to a hospital where the patient is currently having treatment – or has recently completed treatment – may not be the most conducive environment in which to offer complementary therapies. Redler supports this view by stating that 'For some it may be too painful to continually meet up with the staff associated with their illness, reminding them of a situation they are trying to forget'.[5] Complementary therapies may be appropriate in helping patients from diagnosis, throughout periods of adaptation and during terminal phases. Carers, for whom it is also crucial to offer support, may be more inclined to take up services in this type of environment. Therefore, a local community-based service can offer a more relaxed, less clinical environment which is easily accessed by local people. It may also be advantageous to encourage self referral which allows the person to feel a sense of control. A range of complementary therapies should be offered for support, and following explanation and discussion the client should choose a therapy which best suits his/her needs. This approach encourages and can actually enhance self empowerment.

> I've only called in once or twice
> Finding the staff helpful, friendly and nice,
> I heard it was just the right place
> Where people will listen and give you some space.
> The first call is the hardest but it's really up to you,
> If you are able to call in or phone for a chat
> You're trying to help yourself if you cannot do just that.
> The centre there's no doubt will help you to recover,
> After the first step by you they will help you take another.
> I think I've said enough for now, the rest is up to you –
> Pick up the phone and make a call, and find all I've said is true.
>
> *Help Yourself by Hilda Rose (a patient)*

This service can be fully integrated into a palliative day care centre and greatly enhances the holistic support offered to patients (Figure 23.1).

The aim of the therapies in this context would be to:

1. Enhance the relaxation process;
2. Promote a sense of well-being;
3. Act as a pathway to communication;
4. Have a role in symptom control.

Case history

A gentleman with cancer of the colon, with recurrent disease and also a colostomy. In an attempt to control symptoms of nausea, anti-emetic drugs were given via a syringe driver. However, the problem of nausea persisted. He agreed to attend for relaxation and aromatherapy. It was decided that peppermint should be used to settle his stomach and to apply this through hand massage. The next week he reported an ease in feelings of nausea on the evening of treatment and requested it again. The one-to-one patient/therapist intervention gave him the opportunity to discuss frustrations in no longer being able to participate in his interests, and the opportunity to replace this by joining in some diversional therapies ... which he did.

The potential benefits of complementary therapies have yet to be demonstrated scientifically. However, anecdotally there does appear to be evidence that patients

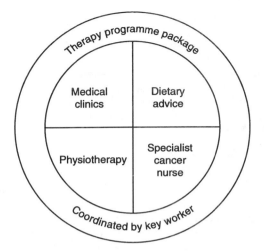

Fig. 23.1 The complementary therapy programme.

report some benefit and Wells (1994) has said that 'complementary therapies did not necessarily need validating by science or medicine. If a patient said that he or she felt better for it, then this was justification for providing it'.[6] Downer *et al.* remark that patient satisfaction with both conventional and complementary therapies was high, and for complementary therapies satisfaction was, '. . . high even without the hoped for anti-cancer effect. Patients reported psychological benefits such as hope and optimism'.[7] The importance of maintaining hope has been well demonstrated. Scanlon in her article on rehabilitation in palliative care asserts that 'Hope is not based on false optimism or benign reassurance, but is built instead on the belief that better days or moments can come in spite of the prognosis'.[8] Complementary therapies can help to alleviate the hopelessness felt by people with life-threatening diseases and help them to have more 'better days and moments'. Hope is important because without its essential quality a person is prevented from living until they die. 'Hope itself is a contagious reality, for without hopefulness of others, it is almost impossible for patients to remain or become hopeful. It is our hopefulness as nurses that is indispensable in palliative caring'.[8] Complementary therapies provide the path to hope which is so essential to patients with life-threatening diseases.

Complementary therapies, especially those such as aromatherapy and reflexology, provide much-needed time for people to be nurtured. A 70-year-old lady, a carer, who had agreed to attend an aromatherapy group session, initially with some reluctance, was heard to comment afterwards: 'I have had time to myself for the first time in my life'.

Setting up a complementary therapy programme in a day centre

Early planning, communication and enlisting the support of other health care professionals certainly pays dividends. The involvement of key people from the primary health care team (such as having a GP as chair of the planning committee) would be an invaluable asset in gaining acceptance. The credibility of the centre could be increased by the service and support of a consultant in palliative care and the team being led by an experienced palliative care specialist such as a Macmillan nurse. The lines of communication between the centre and health care professionals working in both hospital and community settings should be maintained from the earliest stages. One suggestion regarding communication might be to hold an open week prior to commencing services. Another would be to speak to key people in the following areas:

- Local district general hospitals
- The local specialist cancer hospital
- All local GP services.

This initial contact should be followed up by written information.

From opening, regular weekly team meetings should be held and community nurses, dietitians, social workers, etc. should be invited to meet with the team for an informal exchange of ideas and news on a monthly basis and also offer monthly visitors' mornings. Another communication exercise which might be helpful is to invite the more sceptical consultants to join in a complementary therapy session following which conversion may take place!

There are, of course, pitfalls which may be encountered when attempting to incorporate complementary therapies in a palliative day care setting. From professional colleagues, some thoughts which have been articulated include:

1. A distrust of the self-referral policy;
2. Concern and worry regarding patients who might decide to abandon conventional medicine/therapies altogether;
3. A lack of scientifically based research, i.e. double-blind trials;
4. A fear of untrained or under-trained therapists;
5. Professional cynicism regarding the multi-disciplinary approach.

Important considerations in setting up a service

- Space/building
- Surroundings/atmosphere
- Therapists
- Therapies.

Space

Hopefully, the introduction of complementary therapies as part of an holistic service will be successful, so rather than start with one room and then have to expand, 'think big' originally so that time and effort may be put into patient care after the initial, inevitable frustrations of commissioning a purpose-built area. It is important to have individual small counselling and therapy rooms for privacy and quiet. In a study by Wilkinson conducted at the Marie Curie Centre in Liverpool, although 75 per cent of those interviewed considered the facilities 'very satisfactory'[9] the requests for improvements were mainly to do with space and privacy.

Surroundings

The attempted ideal to achieve is a 'home from home' atmosphere and attention to colour and furniture will pay dividends:

> I was amazed at what I saw, not only tasteful decor and furnishings, but a relaxed easy atmosphere. There were no beds, no doctors, no white coats and no obviously sick people ... it was a non-demanding place where I was guided but not looked after ...

Also, attention to the atmosphere and surroundings will be conducive to beginning the process of relaxation.

Therapists

In order to present as much choice as possible it would follow that the number of therapies on offer should be as diverse as possible; but given by whom? One avenue is to employ therapists who are qualified in complementary therapies either on a paid or voluntary basis. However, it may be possible, when appointing health professionals to the team, to employ those with qualifications in the complementary field. The only disadvantage, perhaps, with this is the restriction imposed by the size of the team which, initially, is bound to be small. The team may increase thereby augmenting the choice of therapies on offer. As the number of therapists increases it may be possible to support a member of the professional team to undertake a qualification in one of the complementary therapies such as the Diploma in Aromatherapy who may then lead a therapy team. The use of trained volunteers in the team may be useful. An advantage in widening the network of therapies is that as people are highly individual in the way they relate to others, it is more possible to ensure that team members are available who have different skills and a diversity of approaches. The selection procedure for paid or unpaid non-health professional therapists should ensure that aspects of confidentiality and adherence to standards means that the patient's integrity can be maintained. It is essential to develop a written protocol for all to follow which includes agreement on acceptable qualifications and necessary supervision for staff with minimal training. Recruitment of these therapists is better maintained by word of mouth rather than any advertisement.

Therapies

Some criteria for choosing the therapies offered is essential because of their diversity in number. Availability of therapies may be governed by the qualifications of the staff. This may mean some of the more well-known therapies being offered and these may vary from area to area, and certainly country to country. Fisher and Ward have found 'some intriguing national idiosyncrasies, for example, reflexology is particularly popular in Denmark (39 per cent of complementary medicine users). This relates to the legal situation – in 1981 the Danish High Court ruled that acupuncture is a form of surgery since it pierces the skin. Reflexology which is related to acupuncture does not'.[10] However, account should be taken of the fact that complementary therapies will not suit everyone's needs nor conform to personal views. Some of the reasons for patients' reluctance to take up the complementary therapies on offer include a fear of invasive therapeutic methods coupled with the fact that private space may be infringed upon and the possibility of a patient's distrust of intimate contact with someone who is, as yet, unfamiliar to them. The notion that complementary therapies may be a medium for the person to 'heal themselves' from within has been questioned by some religious bodies and religious consideration should always be kept in the forefront of therapists' minds.

Case history: elderly lady with diagnosis of head and neck tumour

Unfortunately, side-effects of the treatment have caused a degree of deafness and she is also partially sighted. She chooses to have a hand massage with lavender oil. The aim of this treatment is to stimulate her sense of smell as other senses are depleted. The one to one contact allows her to discuss her own agenda; she uses time well, knowing she has the therapist's individual attention. She says she feels more relaxed and comforted at the end of the massage. She looks happy and cheerful as if she has had a special treatment.

There is another dimension to some of these therapies. Touch is intrinsic to the therapeutic process: 'To touch is not a technique: not touching is a technique'.[11] To be touched is a very important part of our interaction with others which involves a communication of love and security with implications for physical survival and emotional self esteem. In *Supportive therapies in health care*, Wells (1994) states that: 'practitioners and clients use reflexology because:

- it is not invasive and there is no perforation of the skin;
- it is inexpensive in equipment and resources, except that of the therapist's time;
- it may become an alternative to medication; as drugs become increasingly expensive costs may be reduced;
- initial effect of relaxation and 'winding down';
- quality of sleep improves, consequently people feel that they will sleep more deeply and are more alert when awake;
- pain and symptoms are relieved where the therapy is appropriately used;
- continuity of care between the client and a regular therapist is felt by both parties to be an advantage;
- many people including the seriously ill, the terminally ill and the elderly, respond appreciatively to touch'.[12]

The services of health professionals who are not full-time members of the team can be bought in and this could have the advantage of improved liaison and communication. A local GP offering sessions of acupuncture and homeopathy may increase the credibility of the service. The increase and growth of a programme which includes complementary therapies may occur through a combination of:

- an increase in therapists (members of the multi-disciplinary team) acquiring extra skills;
- external therapists offering services and then being trained 'in-house';
- patients requesting new therapies.

An example of such growth may be seen from this current programme of activities which grew from initially offering only aromatherapy, relaxation and reflexology (Table 23.1).

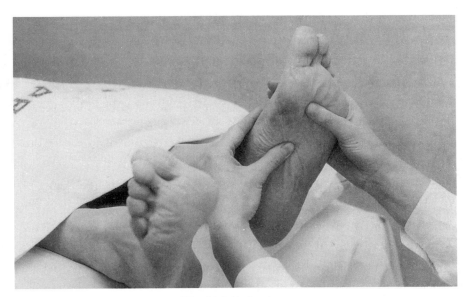

Fig. 23.2 Reflexology.

A balance should be maintained between individual and group therapies to widen the choice. Careful assessment is required to couple the individual needs of patients and carers to the services offered within the ability of a palliative day care. Acknowledgement of the constant interactions between body, mind, emotions and spirit means that continual re-assessment is required.

Table 23.1 Programme of complementary therapies

Mornings	Afternoons
Tuesday	
Reflexology	Reflexology
Painting for pleasure	Tai Chi
Wednesday	
Day care	Acupuncture
Handicrafts	Relaxation
	Homoeopathy
Thursday	
Reflexology	Reflexology
Relaxation	Aromatherapy
	Stress management
Friday	
Individual full body massages and aromatherapy massages	

Problems may be encountered where the demands of the clients exceed the time available. A system should be devised to meet the needs of as many clients within the constraints of time as possible, whilst always maintaining high standards, to satisfy the aim of enhancing the relaxation process and promote a sense of well-being. As a day care patient has said:

> The therapy and relaxation have helped me to help myself. If I had not been able to face my situation, accept it, understand it and put words to the feelings I have been through I don't think I could have coped. It is my life – a very precious life.

In addition to clinical practise the members of the team need to ensure that through explanation and advice both the lay public and health professional colleagues encourage clients to self refer.

What of the future for complementary therapies? We should, perhaps, be considering ways in which all therapies could be better integrated into existing health care practice by the regulation of training, an increase in research and more education. In an ideal world, people could have the benefit of a full, holistic service. As both conventional and complementary treatments aim to secure the well-being and comfort of patients, it would appear that the two traditions should be merged to fully complement patient care and reach the pursued ideal 'something making up a whole' from which people in need would benefit.

References

1. *Collins English dictionary and thesaurus.* London: Harper Collins Publishers, 1992.
2. Wells R, Tschudin V. Preface. In: *Wells' supportive therapies in health care.* London: Ballière Tindall, 1994; 189.
3. Fisher P, Ward A. Complementary medicine in Europe. *BMJ* 1994; **309**: 107.
4. Burke C, Sikora K. Complementary and conventional cancer care: the integration of 2 cultures. *Clin Oncol Roy Coll Radiol* 1993; 5(4): 220–27.
5. Redler N. A triumphant survival, but at what cost? (Meeting the long-term needs of cancer survivors). *Profess Nurse*, December 1994, 169.
6. Wells R, Tschudin V. Preface. In: *Wells' supportive therapies in health care.* London: Ballière Tindall, 1994; 189.
7. Downer SM, *et al.* Pursuit and practice of complementary therapies by cancer patients receiving conventional treatment. *BMJ* 1994; **309**: 86.
8. Scanlon C. Creating a vision of hope: The challenge of palliative care. *Oncol Nurs Forum* 1989; **16**: 491.
9. Wilkinson S. Aromatherapy and massage in palliative care – does it improve patients' quality of life? *Internat J Palliat Nurs* 1995; 1.
10. Fisher P, Ward A. Complementary medicine in Europe. *BMJ* 1994; **309**: 107.
11. Autton N. Touch in counselling and psychotherapy. In: *Touch an exploration.* London: Darton, Longman and Todd, 1989; 89.
12. Lett A. Reflex zone therapy. In: Wells R, Tschudin V, eds. *Wells' supportive therapies in health care.* London: Ballière Tindall, 1994; 189.

24

Postscript

Ronald Fisher

I went into hospital to be cured and almost died.
Then I went into Hospice to die, and lived.

A patient writing in the Washington Post

Efficiency is the order of the day and rightly so, but it must be efficiency with empathy. We must never forget our origins and the basic principles on which the hospice movement was founded. This does not mean, however, that we have to follow too rigidly yesterday's ideas, however relevant they were at the time.

For example, it was said in the 1970s that specialist home care nurses were needed because the district nurses did not have the time or the skills to care for those patients whose cancers had not responded to curative treatment. Likewise, it was said that specialist physicians were needed because effective pain and symptom control was rarely achieved. But that was yesterday. Today the increase in knowledge and the achievements in palliative medicine have boosted the interest and realisation of the importance of effective palliative care.

Specialists do not have the exclusive rights to practice palliative care, but they do have a duty to pass on their expertise to others, and in the works of Derek Doyle[1] to act in a concerted and coordinated way.

There is an innate ability in many of us to give palliative care and that ability can be greatly enhanced by education and training. Derek Doyle, chairman of the European Association for Palliative Care Education Committee, always a strong advocate for further education and training, says that this is not taken seriously enough.[2] Member states of the European Union have recommended that this should be given a high priority, not only for doctors and nurses, but hopefully for others who are involved in community care.

Acting in a concerted and coordinated manner and giving a high priority to education are fine-sounding words. But do we have the leadership to achieve these worthy ideals? We have various associations, professional bodies, Royal Colleges and charities, all involving themselves, but no coordinator, no conductor for our palliative care ensemble.

Professor Hanks in the preface reminds us that there should be emphasis on coordination between the primary care sector and the hospice movement, and that palliative services should be integrated with general practice.

We are in danger of creating a myth that if you are dying from cancer then you have to do it with a specialist nurse. No one knows better than myself the value of the specialist community nurses. They are vital to the service, but then so is the district nurse. Before flooding the market place could we not at least try to enhance the role of the district nurse?

Specialists, consultants, medical directors, experts, call them what you will, are absolutely essential, not only to develop palliative medicine for the good of all, but to be available to give help and advice for those patients with difficult problems.

If it is shown that community nurses can be taught to give effective holistic care, then this should influence the number of specialist nurses needed in the future and be more cost effective.

Our predicament reminds me of the Pirandello play *Six characters in search of an author;*[3] or perhaps since we already have an author in Dame Cicely Saunders we should stretch the analogy and change the title to six (or more) bodies in search of a coordinator.

In Pirandello's play, a rehearsal is in progress when suddenly the stage is invaded by six characters who infiltrate into the company and try to use the rehearsal for their own purposes. They are trying to find their own identity, to see themselves, to justify their existence, to find guidance.

In the foreword to the play Pirandello writes:

When a man lives, he lives and does not see himself.
Well – put a mirror before him and make him see himself in
the act of living.

Or in the act of doing!
Henry Ford once said:

'coming together is a beginning,
keeping together is progress,
working together is success'.

We have begun, we are progressing, but we can be more successful.

So mull over David Clark on 'Whither the hospices'[4] take note of Irene Higginson's contribution in Chapter 10 – and buy a large mirror.

References

1. Doyle D. A time for definition. *J Palliat Med* 1993; 7(4): 253.
2. Doyle D. Education and training in palliative medicine in European Community medicine states. *Europ J Palliat Care* 1994; 1(1): 52–3.
3. Pirandello L. (1867–1936). Italian playwright. Awarded Nobel Prize in 1934.
4. Clark D. Whither the hospices? In: *The future for palliative care – issues of policy and practice*. Buckingham: Open University Press, 1993.

Index